# THE 6 WEEK
# HERBAL
# DETOX
# PLAN

## PETER CONWAY

PIATKUS

For my mother – generous, kind and remarkable –
with all my love

Herbal medicine does not replace normal allopathic treatment.
It is a means of supporting and complementing such medical
treatment. If you have any acute or chronic disease you should
seek medical attention from a qualified doctor. The author and
publisher accept no liability for damage of any nature resulting
directly or indirectly from the application or use of information
in this book.

Copyright © 2003 by Peter Conway

First published in 2003 by
Judy Piatkus (Publishers) Limited
5 Windmill Street
London W1T 2JA
e-mail: info@piatkus.co.uk

**The moral right of the author has been asserted**

*A catalogue record for this book is available from the British Library*

ISBN 0 7499 2324 5

Edited by Matthew Cory
Text design by Jerry Goldie

This book has been printed on paper manufactured with respect for the
environment using wood from managed sustainable resources

Printed and bound in Great Britain by MPG Books Ltd, Bodmin,
Cornwall

# CONTENTS

# Acknowledgements

I would like to thank my teachers in herbal medicine. I am particularly indebted to Kerry Bone and Simon Mills for their work in furthering the modern practice of herbal medicine, or phytotherapy, and I gratefully acknowledge their seminal work *Principles and Practice of Phytotherapy* (*see* Further Reading) which has been a major guide for me and one of the main references used in this book for dosage recommendations. I would like to pay tribute again to Hein Zeylstra, former Principal of the College of Phytotherapy, who died shortly before work on this book began. The memory of his energy, knowledge and wisdom will continue to be an inspiration to me.

To my patients and students I owe an enormous debt – you frequently teach me more than I teach you. At Piatkus I am especially grateful to Sandra Rigby and Anna Crago – your guidance and patience have been hugely valued – and to Penny Philips and my marvellous editor Matthew Cory. I thank Paul Chenery of Rutland Organics for his advice on Chapter 3, though any errors are entirely my own and not his, and Dr Ann Walker of the Department of Human Nutrition at Reading University for so skilfully sharing her knowledge of nutrition and herbal medicine. I am also indebted to Dr Terry Willard of Wild Rose College, Calgary, Canada for teaching me about Syndrome X.

Thank you Morgaine for being passionate, Angelica for being harmonious and Tristan for being simply so much fun – shall we go out and play now?

*Many thanks to: The Anonymous 4 (and Hildegarde of Bingen), David Darling, Keith Jarrett, Orchestra Baobab, Yann Tiersen, The Velvet Underground (via Robert Quine), J.S. Bach, Olivier Messiaen, The Peatbog Faeries, Hilmar Orn Hilmarsson, Sigur Ros and many others for providing the soundtrack to the writing of this book – never forget the healing power of art!*

# Introduction

Detoxification is a fundamental process of cleansing and revitalising. It clears the way to make a new start, but detox is just the beginning of better health...

In this book we will go beyond detox to show you a complete and easy-to-follow approach to improving your health with herbal medicines accompanied by dietary and lifestyle changes.

Herbal medicine is the oldest form of medicine and it is still the commonest form of medicine in use today. Around a quarter of all conventional drugs are derived from medicinal plants and, in fact, the word *drug* itself derives from the Old French word *drogue*, meaning a dried herb.

Conventional medicine in the West evolved out of herbal medicine and up to the 1930s the majority of a doctor's remedies were herbal remedies. The development of the pharmaceutical industry heralded in a new age of synthetic medicines and such new treatments have had major successes, particularly in controlling infectious diseases.

But, there are limits to the scope of conventional drugs. Many common and chronic conditions remain inadequately treated. As the population lives longer, the quality of health we enjoy in our later years is often poor. Another troublesome problem is the diminishing effectiveness of antibiotics. An overfamiliarity with these drugs causes bacteria and other micro-organisms to develop resistance to them, leading to the creation of 'super bugs'.

Over the last few decades there has been a resurgence of interest in herbal medicine. One of the reasons for this is the growing dissatisfaction with the conventional treatment of chronic illness, together with a concern about the toxicity and potential side effects of drugs. We also have an increased desire to exercise greater control over our health and to choose our own path to well-being. In addition, there is a concern that modern medicine focuses too much on the physical body at the expense of our emotional, mental and spiritual make-up. This is accompanied by a growing awareness of green issues which is reflected in a demand for treatments that are more natural and ecological and less technological.

The renaissance of herbal medicine has been backed by rigorous research into herbs and this has provided scientific credibility for plant medicines. In realising that there are limits to high-tech medicine, in some areas we are now returning, quite literally, to the roots of healing. While conventional medicine remains supreme in the initial treatment of emergency conditions, herbal medicine has much to offer in treating the minor to moderate conditions of everyday life.

Another area in which herbal medicine excels, and in which conventional drugs have virtually no role, concerns the enhancement of normal bodily functioning to help us achieve optimum health and prevent future disease taking hold. Conventional medicine only treats illness once it is established, but herbal medicine offers the potential to make disease less likely to occur in the first place. This is the focus of this book – using herbs to prevent illness and to engender optimum health with detox as the key starting point.

Herbal remedies have the power to correct abnormal bodily functions but they can also enhance normal ones. Traditionally, herbs that have this effect have been described as 'tonics'. The beautiful North American herb echinacea (*Echinacea purpurea*) improves the immune response to infection so that when you catch common infections such as colds or flu, they are not as severe and do not last as long as they otherwise would. The humble dandelion root (*Taraxacum officinale*) has a bitter taste that stimulates the gall bladder, stomach, liver and pancreas, resulting in better absorption of nutrients from food, more comfortable bowel movements and increased energy levels.

But herbs do not only work on the physical level. They can also influence our emotional well-being and mental performance. Common oats (*Avena sativa*) have long been used in herbal medicine to nourish and strengthen the nervous system, promoting emotional stability. The root of the herb valerian (*Valeriana officinalis*) quells tension and reduces anxiety. The leaves of the Chinese ginkgo tree (*Ginkgo biloba*) improve circulation to the brain, enhancing concentration and memory.

In *The 6 Week Herbal Detox Plan*, in addition to discovering the best herbs to use to cleanse the body, you will learn about many other herbs that you can incorporate into your daily lifestyle to help you achieve optimum levels of health. These range from the 'super herbs' such as Korean ginseng (*Panax ginseng*) to less known but equally useful herbs such as the remarkable Indian plant ashwagandha (*Withania somnifera*) which has been used in the Middle East to improve the performance of racehorses and has traditionally been said to impart the 'vitality of the horse' to human beings!

In order to provide an accessible way to gain the full benefits of the herbal approach, this book has been devised as a 6-Week Plan. This plan has been designed to enable you to work with the most effective methods and herbs to improve and protect your health.

In **Part I**, we explore the origins, philosophy and practice of herbal medicine, and the specific ways in which herbs influence our health. We look at how we can get the most from using herbs, including practical information on buying, growing and preparing herbs. There is also an introductory overview of the Herbal Detox Plan, which shows how you can begin to transform your health with herbs in just six weeks.

**Part II** describes the three fundamental herbal strategies that everyone can use to achieve better health with herbs. These are:

- Detoxification,
- Antioxidants,
- Adaptogens.

These are looked at in depth, and guidance is given on which herbs to use and how to take them.

The chapters in **Part III** take a detailed look at bodily functioning, system by system, and help to identify the particular herbs that can support you and become your allies in achieving full and radiant health. The chapters cover the:

- Immune system;
- Digestive system;
- Circulatory system;
- Respiratory system;
- Bones, muscles and skin;
- Reproductive system;
- Mind and emotions.

Step-by-step self-help treatment guidelines are provided throughout, in addition to guidance on the individual herbs themselves. Each chapter ends with a profile of the one most versatile and important herb for treating the body system discussed. Finally, in the Appendix, essential information is given about the Syndrome X Diet.

By using the herbs and suggestions contained within *The 6 Week Herbal Detox Plan*, you will find help in achieving deep health, and by integrating medicinal plants into your daily life you will be assisted in sustaining this profound health over the years to come.

In my work as a herbal practitioner, I have seen and enjoyed the improvements that herbs have made in the health of my patients, my family and myself. Generally, some signs of improvement can be expected within six weeks of beginning the treatment and it is possible to achieve extensive health improvements within this time. The sooner you start, the sooner you will begin to feel the healing and invigorating benefits of herbs. It is time to cease to cope and to start to thrive!

To your good health.
Peter Conway
Tunbridge Wells, 2002

# PART I

# Laying the Foundations

# Chapter 1

# INTRODUCING HERBAL MEDICINE

Herbal medicine is a system of medicine that uses plant preparations to promote optimum health and to prevent and treat disease. Many books have been written about the use of herbs to treat established disease, but this book focuses on using herbs to improve our health and prevent disease occurring in the first place.

The role of herbs in preventive medicine has long been valued both as part of our general diet and in specific healing practices. Although in earlier times, people had no conception of bacteria, nonetheless they had developed the knowledge that herbs such as sage, thyme and rosemary – which have antibacterial properties – not only enhanced the flavour of meat, but also helped to prevent it 'going off' and made it less likely to cause sickness.

Herbs were also used in specific healing techniques such as 'spring cleansing' treatments. Our ancestors would have had little fresh fruit and vegetables over the winter, and they relied on dried meat and fruit, tubers and grains – it would have been quite a stodgy diet, although not necessarily unhealthy if supplies were sufficient. During the spring when fresh green plants were coming through again they would use these to help cleanse and rejuvenate their systems. In the West, herbs such as nettles (*Urtica dioica*), cleavers (*Galium aparine*), dandelion (*Taraxacum officinale*) and burdock (*Arctium lappa*) would have been used. The traditional healing combination of dandelion and burdock has continued in use as a popular drink right through to the present day – although it has developed into a fizzy drink that now contains little or no dandelion and burdock. Nettles are rich in iron and stimulate the circulation, cleavers work on a part of the immune system called the lymphatic system, and both dandelion and burdock stimulate liver and bowel functioning. Taken together these herbs help to revitalise the body and they are all still used today by contemporary herbal practitioners, particularly in the treatment of skin and joint disorders.

This is just one example of how herbs are used to support and strengthen the functioning of all the body systems.

## Herbs in Conventional and Complementary Medicine

Many medical disciplines make use of plants in one form or another. Conventional medicine uses isolated active constituents from plants in a purified (usually chemically synthesised) form – for example, the active ingredients in aspirin derive from the herb meadowsweet (*Filipendula ulmaria*) and the bark of the willow tree (*Salix* species). Likewise, aromatherapy uses semi-purified plant products in the form of volatile or essential oils. Aromatherapists mainly apply oils through the skin via massage. There is also a new healing practice called 'aromatic medicine' which uses plant volatile oils internally, by mouth, as well as externally on the skin. This practice is carried out by some doctors (particularly in France) and herbalists, and it is useful for treating infections as it offers an alternative treatment for bacteria and fungi which have grown resistant to antibiotics. Plants in the form of foods and medicines play a major role in nutritional therapy, providing safe and effective healing resources. They also have a role in naturopathy (as part of hydrotherapy treatments), art therapy (as sources of inspiration), meditation (as focal points) and many other healing approaches.

Homoeopathy is one major medical discipline, outside of herbal medicine, that uses plants. There can be confusion about the differences between herbal medicine and homoeopathy. Looking at these differences will help to illustrate some of the key features of each of them.

## Homoeopathy and herbal medicine

Homoeopathy and herbal medicine use plants in very different ways. Herbal medicines are whole plant preparations that contain the full range of a plant's chemical constituents. Imagine that you have some dried peppermint leaves; you put these in a cup, pour on hot water, then leave the mixture to brew for a few minutes. You will find that the hot water becomes coloured, the steam coming off the cup has the scent of peppermint and, when you drink the tea, it has the characteristic taste of peppermint. All these things happen because chemicals in the plant have been released into the hot water.

These chemicals give peppermint several useful actions: it relaxes the digestive system, stimulates the gall bladder, reduces fevers and, when applied externally, has a cooling and pain-relieving effect, particularly useful in treating headaches and insect bites. It also reduces nasal congestion, loosening phlegm when taken as a tea or as a steam inhalation. The point is that peppermint can do all these things because of the chemicals it contains. The way that these chemicals act on the body can be understood by means of conventional pharmacological knowledge.

Homoeopathic remedies also use herbal preparations as a starting point, and unlike herbal medicine, may use animal and mineral parts as well as plants. However these are then diluted to the extent that they may no longer contain any discernible traces of plant or other chemicals. The effects of homoeopathic medicines do not occur as a result of known chemical processes. Homoeopaths contend that the remedies act by means of energetic vibrations that are somehow released or 'potentised' by the practice of diluting and shaking the remedies. This view pushes at the boundaries of current scientific understanding.

Homoeopathic remedies are prescribed according to the doctrine of 'like treating like'. Essentially, the homoeopathic approach is that if a patient has a disease pattern that is similar to the effects of a substance (such as a plant) when taken in excess, then a very small amount of that substance will serve to clear the disease pattern. An example of this is the popular homoeopathic remedy made from the flowers of the herb arnica (*Arnica montana*). Arnica is not used internally as a herbal remedy because it can cause paralysis of muscles, a change in pulse rate, heart palpitations and difficulty breathing. Taken together these symptoms are similar to those experienced in severe shock, and the homoeopathically diluted preparation of arnica is taken by mouth as an emergency treatment for shock. By contrast, herbal medicine applies herbs to achieve specific effects by modifying normal bodily activities.

## Eastern Herbal Medicine

Different cultures have developed their own ways of understanding and using herbs that fit within their particular cultural viewpoints and circumstances. The best known of these include Traditional Chinese Medicine (TCM), and Ayurvedic medicine from India. There are also several lesser known approaches, such as Unani-Tibb medicine (also from India), Maori medicine and Kanpo medicine (from Japan).

TCM uses plant, mineral and animal substances, as well as the ancient practice of acupuncture, to form a comprehensive treatment system. However, TCM practitioners in the West avoid using animal products.

Each indigenous medical system tends to have its own way of describing the potential healing power that can be facilitated in the body. To the Chinese this is Qi (or Chi, pronounced 'chee'), to the Ayurvedic practitioner it is Ojus (or prana, the 'inner air') and to the Western herbal practitioner it is the Vital Force (or *vis medicatrix naturae*, the healing power of nature).

Each system also has its own philosophical and practical concepts and techniques that assist the diagnosis and treatment of disease. Chinese herbal medicine uses plants in accordance with the traditional medical understanding of five elements (*wu xing*), which relates diseases and plant activities to the properties of Wood, Fire, Earth, Metal and Water. The Chinese also look at the dynamic interplay of the forces of Yin and Yang. Yin forces are considered to be sustaining, completing and condensing, whereas Yang forces are expanding, transforming and dispersing – a major aim of TCM is to detect disharmonies between Yin and Yang and then seek to correct them.

Ayurvedic practitioners make reference to the concept of the three bodily humours, or *tridoshas*, which are Vata, Pitta and Kapha. Vata is derived from air and space and is associated with the respiratory system and with movement of the body; Pitta arises from the elements of fire and water and is associated with the activities of the digestive system; Kapha is formed from water and earth and is involved in the production of bodily fluids. Ayurvedic medicine also has an appreciation of the seven fundamental constituents of the body (*dhatus*): chyle, blood, flesh, fat, bone, marrow and semen.

In traditional Eastern systems of herbal medicine the importance of supporting elimination in order to avoid congestion and stagnation of vital energies is stressed. In the context of these approaches detox can be seen as both a physical clearing out of waste products and, on another level, a way of keeping the channels of energy in the body clear so that the life force can flow freely and efficiently.

## Western Herbal Medicine

Western herbal medicine is a more broken tradition than that of TCM and Ayurveda. Certainly, in the British Isles traditional medicine was taught orally and little was written down that directly describes the medical concepts of our ancestors. However, there are a few interesting leads, including the writings of the

Welsh 'Physicians of Myddfai' from the eighteenth century, which are thought to hark back to a much earlier indigenous practice of medicine which today we would describe as an holistic approach to healing. Over time, oral knowledge was sidelined by the development of a conventional medical establishment based on the approaches of influential medical schools such as those in Paris, Montpellier, Leiden and, later, Edinburgh, and these would rarely have given credence to local folk medicine practices. Also, changes in the dominant religion often led to the prohibition of traditional medical activities, which were viewed as superstitious at best; this was particularly the case in the seventeenth century in Europe.

Nonetheless, we do know a great deal about the dominant Western medical theory of antiquity. This is the concept of the four humours and their related elements and temperaments.

| Humour | Element | Temperament |
|---|---|---|
| Yellow bile | Fire | Choleric |
| Blood | Air | Sanguine |
| Phlegm | Water | Phlegmatic |
| Black bile | Earth | Melancholy |

For example, people of a melancholic constitution were said to tend towards having dry and cold skin, a slender build, slow pulse and pale urine. Emotionally they were thought to be despondent and sad, and to be loners prone to fearfulness, jealousy and strong ambitions. On a more positive note the melancholic is the intellectual, contemplative character who may achieve great wisdom.

In illness a melancholic picture was associated with an excess of black bile. This is a cold, dry humour that needs to be reduced by the application of herbs with opposing qualities – in this case, heating and moistening. An increase in black bile was connected with excessive cold in the body, or too much heat in the liver, or yet again with weakness of the spleen, which was the 'seat of melancholy' according to the herbalist Culpepper. The melancholic disease state could be tackled by attempting to clear the accumulation of black bile by cleansing or 'purging' the spleen and liver with herbs such as fumitory (*Fumaria officinalis*) and wormwood (*Artemisia absinthium*).

The approach of the four humours, which combines a consideration of the physical, emotional and spiritual aspects of the individual with treatment based on a sophisticated understanding of the way in which herbs act on the body, still has much to teach us today. Insofar as the theory and practice of the four humours concerns itself partly with clearing the excessive build-up of particular material substances (the humours themselves) within the body we can see it as a complex traditional detox methodology.

This scheme, elucidated by the 'father of medicine' Hippocrates (c.460–377BC) and later followers, especially Galen (c.129–216AD), provided the main framework for the diagnosis of disease and the application of herbal remedies in the West by the medical profession for around 2,000 years.

## Balancing the body and mind

There are many similarities between the different traditional ways of understanding health and the functions of the body. The Chinese Yin/Yang theory relates in part to the Western desire to balance activity and rest, or exertion and relaxation. Five element theory has correspondences with the four humours and the *tridoshas*. A common thread is the concept of achieving equilibrium, or what might described in medical terms today as 'homoeostasis'. Homoeostasis may be a misleading word because our internal states are never static, but always changing depending on our circumstances and requirements. Harmony arises when we achieve a dynamic balance on all four levels of our being – our physical, emotional, mental and spiritual functioning. Disharmony and disease arise when there is an extreme of activity in any one single area, so losing sight of the centre where health is to be found. The essential purpose of herbal medicine is to identify areas of imbalance and use herbs to steer the individual back to the central point of equilibrium and optimum functioning.

## Western Herbal Medicine Today

Nowadays we have the advantage of being able to combine a conventional modern medical understanding of anatomy and physiology with an approach that is both holistic (considering and treating the whole person) and naturopathic (working with, rather than against, nature). Since I am trained as a Western herbalist, this book follows the Western approach, but I use herbs from all around the world and you will find herbs mentioned from areas such as China, Asia and Africa, as well as Europe and North America.

Herbal medicine in the West is evolving and its practice is modified as fresh research throws light on the best ways to use herbs to achieve optimal results. Research has helped us to a better understanding of how herbs work, how to classify them, and how to know which herbs are the best for particular conditions. Importantly, it has also enhanced our awareness of safety issues in herbalism.

This new science-based practice of herbal medicine is sometimes referred to as phytotherapy – *phyto* is Greek for 'plant'. But herbal medicine is not only a science, it is also an art. In order to practise herbal medicine it is necessary to have a scientific appreciation of the way the body works and of the constituents and actions of plants on the body. However, it is also important to apply the artistic qualities of intuition and creativity in assessing patients and developing prescriptions in order to arrive at a full understanding of the patient and their treatment needs. The modern herbal practitioner, or phytotherapist, combines both art and science, intuition and rationalism in helping to support the health of individuals.

Many of the earliest written records of herbal medicine, such as the Egyptian Ebers papyrus (c.1550BC – the oldest surviving medical text) contain extensive lists of plants and their medicinal uses. The great names in the history of medicine – Hippocrates, Galen,

Dioscorides and Avicenna – were all herbalists. It is a practice of medicine that extends across all cultures and throughout history. People once developed their understanding of plants' healing powers through trial and error, then by more structured experimentation. Classification of herbal actions was developed and based on sensory and clinical experience – herbs were categorised as being heating or cooling, moistening or drying, bitter or sweet, stimulating or relaxing. With the development of the sciences of chemistry and pharmacology, it has been possible to examine the constituents of herbs and categorise them chemically.

Today there is access to a large number of older herbal texts, such as John Gerard's *Herbal or General Historie of Plantes* (1597), and more recent important works such as the writings of the American Physiomedicalist and Eclectic herbal physicians from the beginning of the twentieth century, and Maud Grieve's influential *A Modern Herbal* (1931). In addition, there is a growing number of research papers, looking at all aspects of herbal practice. The modern herbal practitioner is now able to work in a way that combines the best of herbal medicine's past with the insights gained from present developments.

## National standards

Until the early twentieth century, botany remained a core subject in medical schools and the majority of drugs used by trained physicians were of plant origin. Formal training of herbal practitioners and medical herbalists also developed, although on a relatively small scale. The National Institute of Medical Herbalists was founded in 1864 and has been the main body overseeing the herbal profession in the UK ever since, promoting the establishment of training courses as one of its core activities. Nonetheless, the herbal profession in the UK is still quite small, although with six degree courses in herbal medicine available at UK universities (at the time of writing), it is growing rapidly. In the rest of Europe, herbal medicine is either still practised on a folk basis or used as a tool by conventional doctors. In France, medicine of any description can only be practised by qualified medical doctors, but there is a large demand for the herbal remedies which are available from pharmacies. Several French doctors do practise herbal medicine alongside conventional medicine; amongst these Christian Duraffourd and Jean-Claude Lapraz have been particularly influential in their work and writings. In Germany, most doctors prescribe herbal medicines in addition to conventional drugs, while in the US herbal medicines are mainly prescribed by qualified naturopaths although there is also a small group of herbal practitioners.

## Self-treatment

Herbal medicine is both a recognised professional discipline as well as being a group of remedies available over-the-counter for self-treatment. This situation is similar to that existing in conventional medicine where some drugs are available freely from pharmacies and others only on prescription following a consultation with a doctor. For minor problems, such as coughs and headaches, it is appropriate to go to the pharmacy and buy a short-term treatment, but for a more severe or unusual problem it is preferable to see a doctor. In a similar way, you might go to a pharmacy or health shop to obtain herbs for simple problems, but consult a professional herbal practitioner for a more difficult condition.

As an alternative approach, you might wish to take herbs when you are feeling quite well in order to enhance and protect your health. You could certainly consult a herbal practitioner for advice on how to go about this, but this is an area where this book can be an invaluable guide to how you can integrate herbs into your daily lifestyle as a positive health strategy.

Beginning with detox as a first important step, this book will show you how to work with the key herbal health strategies in achieving a higher level of health. Throughout the book guidance will be given about which specific herbs you can choose that will suit your personal needs.

This book discusses the use of gentle but effective herbs suitable for self-use in the home. Stronger herbs should only be taken on the advice of a herbal practitioner following a full detailed consultation.

# Chapter 2

# PEOPLE AND PLANTS

We could not live without plants. All animal life depends on the ability of plants to convert the sun's energy into products that we can use to sustain ourselves. Plants provide us with the basics we need for survival – food, shelter, clothing and much more besides, including medicines. We depend on plants to prevent the earth from eroding and to keep it fertile, and we need them to regulate and maintain our atmosphere. The relationship we have with plants is an intimate one; it is also, when we consider our use of plants as medicines, a healing relationship.

## Preserving our Relationship with Plants

Our relationship with plants tends to be an unequal one. We need plants but they can survive very well without our presence on this planet and we cause many to be threatened with extinction. One of the key issues in herbal medicine today is conservation – not just the protection of known medicinal plants but of all plants.

Many plants, such as those from the world's rainforests and other remote or inaccessible regions, have not yet been studied for their therapeutic activity and it is probable that there is a vast number of plant remedies out there that we do not yet know about or understand. Some of these remedies are already known to indigenous peoples and this is only one reason why we need to protect their societies and their wisdom. Of course, plants have many other attributes beyond medical activity and no plant should be neglected just because we have yet to find a practical way of using it to help ourselves.

As individuals we can redress the balance in our relationship with plants and start repaying some of the debt we owe them by taking plant conservation seriously and avoiding buying products that are made at the expense of our planet's flora.

We can also exercise caution about the potential benefits of genetic modification of plants. There is some evidence showing that GMOs (genetically modified organisms) can cross-pollinate with wild plants, which may include medicinal herbs, growing in their vicinity. We do not yet know what results this new inter-action might bring about but there is concern that muddying the plant gene pool in this way could have potentially catastrophic effects. As a herbal practitioner my primary anxiety over this issue is that strains of medicinal plants might develop that are either rendered inactive by the influence of GMOs or, worse still, are changed in a way that causes them to produce toxic rather than healing constituents.

One of the great things about herbal medicine is the overlap between the use of plants as foods and plants as medicines, indicating the truly natural and benign character of the healing interaction between people and plants. Hippocrates said, 'Let food be your medicine and medicine be your food'.

## Plant Chemicals – What They Can Do For Us

Primary plant constituents include two forms of nutrients: macro-nutrients, such as fats, carbohydrates and proteins, and micronutrients, such as vitamin C, zinc and selenium.

These have both nutritional and therapeutic activity. However, it is a group of plant products known as 'secondary metabolites' that is considered to provide the more specifically medicinal, non-nutrient actions of herbal remedies. In practice, though, the line between a nutrient and a medicine is often blurred.

Secondary metabolites were once considered to be solely waste products as far as the plant was concerned. Research has since shown that many of these products have a specific function to play, although a precise understanding of these roles is still developing. It seems that many of the metabolites that we use to improve our health also play a part in the plant's health, particularly in areas such as fighting infection, sealing wounds and regulating hormonal functions.

When we take a herbal medicine, it is the secondary metabolic constituents within the plant that interact with and cause changes within our own cells, thus leading to therapeutic effects. Some examples of these constituents are described below.

## Alkaloids

These are nitrogen-bearing plant products that are often highly toxic but can have very rapid and powerful healing effects when used with care. Alkaloid-rich herbs are often of value in treating severe or emergency conditions, and have several beneficial properties, which include:

- Relieving pain;
- Lowering blood pressure;
- Opening up the airways (bronchodilator);
- Treating infections and cancers.

Alkaloids from the opium poppy (*Papaver somniferum*) such as morphine are well known and are used in many very effective painkillers still used widely today in conventional medicine. Alkaloids used in herbal medicine include those in thornapple (*Datura stramonium*) used to treat asthma, and the Chinese herb Ma huang (*Ephedra sinica*) used to treat allergic disorders. Alkaloid-rich herbs should only be taken on the advice of a herbal practitioner.

## Flavonoids

This group of chemicals usually occurs attached to sugars as glycosides (*see* below). Flavonoids tend to be yellow pigments (*flavus* is the Latin for yellow). Anthocyanins give the red, violet and blue-black colours in flowers and fruits. Flavonoids appear to play several important roles in plants, including regulating growth, protecting them from harmful UV radiation and providing defence against infection. In humans they act as strong antioxidants, stabilising cell membranes and preventing damage to cellular contents. They help to improve the condition of the heart and circulation and they protect us against the effects of environmental stress. Flavonoids are present in herbs such as hawthorn leaves, flowers and berries (*Crataegus* species), which are used to treat the heart and circulatory system, and Baical skullcap root (*Scutellaria baicalensis*), which is used to treat allergies, inflammation and high blood pressure.

Fruits rich in flavonoids include cherries, oranges, blueberries, blackcurrants and red and yellow peppers.

## Glycosides

A glycoside is any plant chemical that has a sugar attached to it. When swallowed the glycoside is broken down so the sugar is separated from the active plant chemical, which then goes on to exert its effects. A group of glycosides that has strong effects on the heart is known as 'cardiac glycosides'; these include lily of the valley leaves (*Convallaria majalis*), which are used by herbal practitioners to treat heart failure. Some glycosides are strong laxatives; they occur in herbs such as the tree cascara sagrada (*Rhamnus purshiana*), which is a very effective detox herb for the bowel but should be avoided during pregnancy as it can have a stimulant effect on the pregnant uterus.

## Gums

Gums are produced by plants to plug wounds, sealing them off from infection. Herbal gums include gum arabic (*Acacia senegal*) and are used for many purposes such as soothing coughs. In medicinal plants, gums are often found in complexes mixed with oils and resins (*see* below) since these constituents normally tend to bind together.

## Mucilages

Mucilage preparations have a soothing effect on the body's internal lining (mucous membranes) and externally on the skin. One of the most noted herbal mucilages is the powdered inner bark of the slippery elm tree (*Ulmus rubra*). Mucilaginous pastes are wonderful for coating inflamed and sore areas of the digestive system in conditions such as heartburn (reflux oesophagitis) and colitis. Mucilaginous teas, such as those made from marshmallow leaves (*Althaea officinalis*), or mullein leaves and flowers (*Verbascum thapsus*), are excellent for soothing the airways in dry sore coughs.

## Napthoquinones

These are quinone-based chemicals that can be antibacterial and antifungal. They include juglone from the leaves of the English walnut (*Juglans regia*) and butternut (*Juglans cinerea*) and lapachol from the amazing South American tree pau d'arco (*Tabebuia* species), which has immune boosting and anticancer properties.

## Resins

Resins are common in conifers such as pine trees. Frankincense (*Boswellia sacra*) and myrrh (*Commiphora molmol*) are resins and, in common with most resins, this famous pair are aromatic (the resin contains a volatile oil). Resins are highly antimicrobial – for instance, mastic from the mastic tree (*Pistacia lentiscus*) is effective against the bacteria that cause stomach ulcers (*Helicobacter pylori*). The resin from marigold flowers (*Calendula officinalis*) is antifungal and stimulates the immune system. Resins do not dissolve in water but will mix readily with alcohol. This makes them ideal to prescribe as tinctures (water/alcohol preparations).

## Saponins

Saponins are bitter tasting, sometimes toxic to animals, and have been used as fish poisons. As medicines, horse chestnut seeds (*Aesculus hippocastanum*) are used to improve the integrity of the walls of veins, making them useful for treating varicose veins and haemorrhoids, and lime flowers (*Tilia* species) help to lower blood cholesterol levels. A group of specialised saponins have 'adaptogenic' qualities that improve our physical stamina and mental performance. These are found in Korean ginseng (*Panax ginseng*). There is much more on this in the chapter on adaptogens (*see* pages 95–108).

## Tannins

Tannins bind proteins and pull animal membranes tightly together, acting as an astringent agent. They are present in many plants; notable sources of medicinal tannins include oak bark (*Quercus robur*) and witch hazel bark and leaves (*Hamamelis virginiana*). Tannins bind secretions and are of value in treating diarrhoea, dysentery and wounds. They staunch bleeding and bind skin proteins together, very quickly creating a leathery scar. They are also useful for heavy menstrual bleeding and in reducing inflammatory swellings, and they can be antibacterial and antiviral.

Tannins are divided into two groups: condensed (only partially soluble in water and alcohol), and hydrolysable (dissolving easily in water). Condensed tannins can be excellent antioxidants, offering profound health benefits due to their ability to reduce cellular damage. Both green tea and red wine are good sources of beneficial condensed tannins.

A class of condensed tannins called oligomeric procyanidins (OPCs), also known as pycnogenols, possesses potent antioxidant activity helping to promote a healthy vascular system. OPCs are present in maritime pine bark (*Pinus pinaster*), grape vine leaves (*Vitis vinifera*) and hawthorn trees (*Crataegus* species).

The drawback with some tannins is that they can bind with nutrients in the diet, or other herbs in a prescription, thus reducing their availability to the body. It is not a good idea to drink too much strong tea as this can lead to nutritional depletion.

## Volatile oils

Volatile oils (also known as essential oils) are complex aromatic compounds. They are responsible for the scents of herbal medicines such as cinnamon bark (*Cinnamomum zeylanicum*), lemon balm leaves (*Melissa officinalis*) and chamomile flowers (*Matricaria recutita*). While pure distilled volatile oils are used in aromatic medicine and aromatherapy, in herbal medicine they are usually left within the original plant part containing them – such as the leaf or flower. Volatile oils can have many actions including being antimicrobial, relaxant to the muscles, stimulating circulation and boosting the immune system.

# The Actions of Herbs

Looking at herbs in terms of their active chemical groups as above is just one way of classifying herbs.

## Herbal safety

One broad categorisation of herbal actions could be made in terms of their safety risk. We can class herbs as being:

- **Gentle** – very unlikely to cause any adverse effects;
- **Moderate** – potentially causing some mild side effects such as stomach irritation;
- **Strong** – capable of causing unpleasant side effects such as palpitations or vomiting;
- **Toxic** – liable to cause severe or lasting damage to the human body.

The vast majority of medicinal herbs can be placed in the gentle to moderate category and these are the focus of this book.

## Therapeutic effects

A more detailed classification can be made by looking at the specific therapeutic actions of herbs – the precise influence that the herb has on the body. A number of terms are used here, many of which are familiar from their use in conventional medicine, such as 'anti-inflammatory' but others, such as 'nervine', are rarely used outside of herbal medicine. Most herbs have more than one action; so, for example, chamomile (*Matricaria recutita*) is anti-inflammatory, anti-spasmodic, slightly sedative, antibacterial, regulates stress and is wound healing. It is one of the joys of herbal medicine that one herb can do so much.

## Energetic activities

Traditionally herbs were classified according to their physical and sensory characteristics and by what might be called their 'energetic' activities. This kind of classification continues today in approaches such as traditional Chinese medicine. The Chinese system contains the concept of dividing herbs into five tastes:

- Salty,
- Sour,
- Bitter,
- Sweet,
- Pungent (or acrid).

The pungent category is interesting because it does not correspond to a modern understanding of taste – it refers to the raw, hot, penetrating taste of spices such as chilli, ginger, and uncooked garlic and onions. The ways in which herbs stimulate our taste buds have healing effects on the body. For instance, most of the adaptogenic herbs (*see* chapter 7) have a sweet taste and the bitter herbs (*see* chapter 9) have profound effects on the functioning of the liver, gall bladder and digestion. In TCM there is also a sixth 'non-taste' category of 'bland' (tasteless) herbs.

'Energetically' herbs can be classified in other ways, such as by their influence on the temperature of the body or on its fluids and secretions. For example, herbs may be described as being heating or cooling, moistening or drying. Energetic observations about herbs generally derive from extended clinical experience in applying herbs to treat conditions and they can be of great practical value to the herbalist in day-to-day practice.

# Herbal Healing Strategies

With so many herbs to choose from, and many ways in which they might be used, the herbal practitioner needs to decide which to use in any given case. There are a number of key herbal treatment strategies for promoting optimum health and some of the most useful of these are described below. Three of the most important strategies are considered in depth in separate chapters later in this book; these are:

- Detoxification (*see* chapter 5);
- Herbal antioxidants (*see* chapter 6);
- Herbal adaptogens (*see* chapter 7).

Many of the following strategies overlap with each other but they are all working towards the goals of aiding healing, promoting the regeneration of the body and engendering sensations of improved well-being. By using these approaches to improving health, it is often possible to improve substantially the way we feel and how the body functions.

## Restoring the vital force

It is important to nurture, support and restore the vital force when this becomes depleted. This is easy to say but often more difficult to achieve. One needs to identify the areas of health that are weakened and then seek to strengthen them. As you follow the Herbal Detox Plan, this book will help you to identify the areas of your own health that need to be worked on. The vital force can be seen as our sense of energy, vitality and positivity. When we have lots of energy and feel positive and in control, it is possible to live life with purpose and pleasure; conversely, when we feel tired and low it is hard to achieve worthwhile goals and to enjoy life. The vital force is nourished by good sleep, a balanced diet and an enthusiastic, creative mental attitude.

## Promoting equilibrium

Health can be defined as balance and the achievement of equilibrium is the main goal for those pursuing optimum health. Herbalists seek to correct the extreme states that can affect the body's organs, tissues, secretions, or vital functions, and which can 'knock us off balance'. In assessing an individual's state of health, the herbal practitioner will ask questions such as:

- Are the muscles too relaxed or contracted?
- Are the nerves too stimulated or sedated?
- Is the circulation too forceful or weak?
- Is the skin too dry or oily?

By identifying whether there is an excess or deficiency in any particular aspect of the body's function, it is possible to use remedies with an opposing or redressing force to bring that aspect closer to a point of balance.

## Supporting self-healing

It is a fundamental principle of herbal medicine that the body has innate self-healing mechanisms that can be stimulated and supported by the use of herbal remedies. These self-healing mechanisms include the ability of the immune system to neutralise infective organisms, and the capacity of cells and tissues to heal and regenerate themselves, so healing wounds and restoring functions.

## Optimising the performance of individual organs

Some herbs appear to have an affinity for certain tissues, organs or systems, improving their performance. These herbs have been known as 'tonics'. There is no equivalent concept in conventional medicine and this is an important distinguishing feature of herbal medicine. Herbal tonics are given to sustain and enhance particular parts of the body, often as preventive medicines in the absence of any established disease. An example is the use of the hawthorn tree (*Crataegus* species) to support the functions of the heart and circulation. This traditional heart tonic is of immense value today when the commonest cause of death in the developed world is cardiovascular disease.

## Focusing on retention and elimination

It could be said that 'we are what we absorb, not what we eat.' Absorption of nutrients is vitally important to our health and there are herbs that can help this process. Just as important as what we absorb, though, is what we eliminate. By working on the main channels of elimination we can use herbs to keep the body free of congestion. Chapter 5 explores detoxification of these channels (bowel, liver, kidneys, skin, lungs and lymphatic system) in detail.

## Treating the body as a whole

Herbal medicine is a holistic medicine. Consideration should always be given to working on all four levels of human experience. This means paying attention to the physical, emotional, mental and spiritual dimensions of our nature. While herbal medicine can work on all of these levels (though only to a limited extent on the spiritual level), it is not only about giving herbal remedies, but also deals with advising on matters such as diet and lifestyle. It may also be necessary to use other types of medicine or different healing techniques in addition to herbal medicine to treat a particular set of personal health circumstances effectively and to focus on the spiritual level.

# Safety First

It is important to remember that herbs are not invariably an influence for positive change in the body. Just because plants are natural does not mean that they are always safe for us to use. Several medicinal plants used by herbal practitioners have what is called a 'narrow therapeutic window'. This means that the therapeutic dose at which the herb can be given to provide healing benefits is very close to the dose at which the plant can cause toxic damage instead. Such herbs are useful in the hands of an experienced practitioner, often providing rapid and strong results when they are needed in acute or emergency situations, but they should not be used by an untrained person. Any potential safety concerns regarding the herbs covered in this book will be explored as we go along.

While herbal medicine can achieve deep healing with few or no side effects, it is as well to be aware that there are some risks to consider with some herbs, and some people need to take more care with herbs than others. Throughout this book it is indicated where caution should be observed before considering taking a particular herb.

## Groups at increased risk

Though herbal medicine can be used to treat all people of all ages, caution should be exercised in those groups of people who are most vulnerable – children, the elderly, and women who are pregnant or breast-feeding. Particular care needs to be taken if you have a significant medical condition or if you are taking conventional medication prescribed by your medical practitioner.

## Inappropriate herbs

There is a potential for some herbs to make some conditions worse. For example, if you have a situation where the circulatory system is overstimulated, as in cases of high blood pressure, it is inappropriate at the very least, and may be definitely harmful, to take herbs

25

such as Korean ginseng (*Panax ginseng*), which may further stimulate the circulation. It this situation it may be appropriate and beneficial to take herbs that relax and sedate the circulatory system, such as hawthorn (*Crataegus species*).

## Interaction with conventional drugs

There is a potential for some herbs to interact negatively with some conventional drugs. The more vital the need for your conventional medicine, the more caution should be exercised in using herbal medicine. If you are taking drugs that are crucial to your health, such as strong anticoagulants or immunosuppressants, you should have an extremely cautious approach to taking herbs, only doing so with the express approval of your prescribing physician and on the advice of an experienced herbal practitioner. In general, it is wise to check with your doctor and with a qualified herbal practitioner if you have any concerns at all about whether herbal medicine might be right for you in your circumstances.

While no form of treatment is entirely risk free, herbal medicine offers a substantially safer form of therapy than conventional medicine. It is a question of horses for courses – conventional medicine offers massive benefits in the treatment of severe and life-threatening diseases, where the risks from the drugs and other treatments used are far outweighed by the benefits that the treatment brings. Similarly, herbal medicines offer huge advantages in promoting optimum health and in helping to prevent serious disease that far outweigh the minor or rare side effects that some people might experience with certain herbs.

I always say to my students that one of the great things about herbal medicine is that we can get to know our remedies intimately by taking them ourselves, by tasting and experiencing them. Nonetheless, always remember that herbs are powerful healing substances that should be treated with respect.

# Chapter 3

# GETTING THE MOST FROM YOUR HERBAL DETOX PLAN

This chapter deals with the practical aspects of using herbal medicines to improve your health. It provides advice on how to:

- Choose the best-quality herbs;
- Grow, harvest and store herbs;
- Make herbal preparations and how to take them.

## Choosing the Best-quality Herbs

The better the quality of the herbs you use, the better will be the results for your health. Most people buy their herbs from pharmacies or health shops, but a growing number of supermarkets and other outlets are now stocking herbal products. A good way to ensure that you are getting top-quality herbs and herbal preparations is to use a specialist mail order company. Accessing good-quality herbs is often a problem; by and large the suppliers who provide the professional herbal practitioner do not sell their products direct to the public. However, there are some reliable companies that do sell to the public (*see* Resources, page 268).

There are many different kinds of herbal preparations available. I recommend that for self-treatment it is best to use loose dried herbs and make them up into teas. The following advice and tips will help you to select herbs that are likely to be of medicinal quality – and therefore likely to work!

## Herbal quality

There are a number of factors that influence how effective a herbal medicine is likely to be. These include:

- The quality of the plant seed, the place where the plant was grown, the type of soil, the sunlight and rainfall levels, whether the plant was wild-grown or cultivated and, if cultivated, what farming method was used;

- How and when the plant was harvested, how it was dried or prepared and how it was stored;

- How the plant was transported to the point of sale and how it was kept while awaiting sale;

- How old the plant material is (that is to say how long it is since the plant was harvested), since deterioration of the plant's constituents will occur over time.

### Organic v non-organic

When buying herbs you should establish whether they were organically or conventionally grown. Levels of active constituents may be very good in herbs grown either way, but organically grown herbs are more likely to be rich in important nutrients. Crucially, organic herbs will contain no agrochemical pesticides, artificial growth promoters or herbicides. These conventional farming chemicals can cause adverse health effects and have no place in herbal medicine. Also, they upset the natural cycle of life in the soil. It is wise to use organic herbs where possible.

### Genetically modified organisms (GMOs)

The impact that GMOs might have on our well-being is not clear. In some ways we are all participants in a huge experiment. We do know that GM crops can have an adverse effect on our environment by spreading mutated pollen across the countryside, with potentially devastating effects on indigenous plants. To my mind, this is reason enough to avoid GM plants and campaign against GMO technology. Certainly, we do not know how GM herbs might affect our health and so it would be wise to avoid them. The main focus of genetic modification so far has been on food crops rather than herbs, but the genetic manipulation of herbs is beginning to happen and we need to beware of it.

## Wild v cultivated herbs

There is a myth that herbs grown undisturbed in their natural wild habitat are always going to be better than those grown in cultivation. This need not be the case if herbs are cultivated in a sympathetic way in optimum conditions. Where care has been taken to address the plants' growing environment and husbandry needs, cultivated herbs may often be more effective than wild herbs. Well-grown organically cultivated herbs should be used in preference to wild herbs since the latter may be harvested unsustainably, thus leading to conservation dangers.

The line between wild and cultivated herbs can be blurred. I know a grower in Canada who bought a suitably positioned piece of woodland to cultivate Canadian (American) ginseng (*Panax quinquefolius*) and who replicated the wild environment that the plant would naturally experience, leading to the production of medicinal plants of the very highest quality.

## Standardised extracts

Many people see standardised herbal extracts as offering guaranteed quality and efficacy, and a large number of products are marketed with this claim. Unfortunately, things are not that straightforward. A standardised extract is essentially a herbal product that specifies the level of one or more particular active constituents. The implication is that if you have enough of the active constituent/s then the product will definitely achieve the desired results. Such reasoning is the basis of conventional chemical pharmacy, but herbal medicine is rather more subtle.

For many medicinal plants we simply do not know what the main useful active constituents are; plants contain hundreds of chemical compounds and it can be a complex process to unravel which ones are more important than others. Even a widely used herb such as valerian (*Valeriana officinalis*), which has been extensively studied, is still poorly understood in terms of which components should be standardised for.

A further layer of complexity is added when we take into account that it is not only a question of whether there is enough of the main active constituents, but also of the ratio between these and secondary constituents in the plant. This is something that is not understood very well, and perhaps never will be.

A problem can arise with standardised extracts when the content of a strong active constituent is artificially manipulated in the herbal product by adding a purified extract of the desired compound, leading to a level that is not counterbalanced by sufficient levels of other naturally occurring substances in the original plant material. This situation can be potentially dangerous and could, theoretically, make a standardised product more harmful than a non-standardised one. This has led to questions being asked about the safety of some standardised herbs, such as St John's wort (*Hypericum perforatum*) and kava (*Piper methysticum*), two herbs which are considered by herbalists to be very safe when used as non-standardised traditional herbal preparations.

Thankfully, there is a middle ground. It is possible to standardise herbs without artificially manipulating them. This can be done by comparing different batches of particular plants for their active constituent levels (where a particularly active constituent is known). Some batches may have higher levels than considered optimal and some lower; these can then be blended to achieve a specific overall level, thereby guaranteeing that the constituents will be present in harmonious ratios. This type of standardisation is often called 'holistic standardisation' and is the type to be preferred.

Nature is a great chemist, and my advice is to focus less on standardised products for home use, instead ensuring that you have well-grown herbs produced under optimum conditions as these are likely to have the right natural profile of constituents.

## Following your nose – using analeptic testing

In looking to maintain quality control, herbal companies have access to a number of technical resources such as high-performance liquid chromatography (HPLC) to examine the chemical constituents of the plant and check for microbiological contamination. Do read product labels and brochure details to see if manufacturers employ these useful (though limited) aids to ensuring safe and effective products.

When using mainly dried herbs, it is possible to use 'analeptic' tests. All this means is that you can use your senses to check the plants' quality. Analeptic tests are the sort that have been used for thousands of years in the wine trade and by fresh food buyers, using the senses of sight, smell, touch and taste to check the quality of natural products.

**Sight** Does the herb have a good natural vibrant colour or does it look faded or, less commonly, artificially brightened? For example, dried nettle leaves (*Urtica dioica*) should be a rich dark green; dried marigold flowers (*Calendula officinalis*) should be a scintillating golden orange colour.

Does the herb look wilted, stretched or mouldy? Are there any signs of extraneous matter in the sample and is there any evidence that the plant has been nibbled by insects?

**Smell** Does the plant smell fresh and uncontaminated, or does it smell musty or old? If it is a plant smell that you are familiar with, such as peppermint (*Mentha piperita*), does the smell match your memory of what it should be like? With a strongly aromatic herb such as lavender (*Lavandula angustifolia*), is the smell as potent as you would expect, or is it faded or absent, suggesting that the crucial volatile oils have evaporated away? Is the smell too harsh and chemical, suggesting that an artificial scent has been added? Even herbs that do not have strong scents, such as dandelion leaf (*Taraxacum officinale*), should still smell pure, earthy and natural.

**Touch**  Do dried herbs feel dry, clean and vital, or are they damp, bendy and puffy? Dried herbs should generally feel crisp and brittle, and snap cleanly. Fresh herbs should feel springy and resilient to the touch.

**Taste**  Does the plant taste as you would expect it to or is it weak, musty or artificial? Whether a herb tastes pleasant or not is really in the tongue of the beholder. Many herbs are quite bitter and this is a taste that many in the West are unfamiliar with or find difficult.

# Growing, Harvesting and Storing Herbs

Not everyone will want to grow their own herbs, but it is an enjoyable, easy and economic way of ensuring you have access to high-quality fresh herbs. The best herbs to grow for fresh use are the culinary herbs such as sage, chives, parsley, thyme, oregano, rosemary and basil, but you can also grow a wide range of more specifically medicinal herbs if you feel so inclined.

In botanical terms, herbs are plants where the parts above ground die back to ground level each autumn. In these terms, shrubs such as rosemary and sage are not herbs, and trees such as elder and hawthorn certainly are not! The medical definition of a herb is, however, rather broader and encompasses any plant with medicinal activity – shrubs, trees and all.

## Growing

It is beyond the scope of this book to go into great detail, but the most important thing to say is that growing most herbs is easy – many herbs are considered weeds because they are so hardy and propagate so effortlessly. It is wonderful to grow culinary herbs in terracotta pots or in window boxes for use in the kitchen and, if you have the space, useful medicinal herbs can be grown in the garden. When planning which herbs to grow, look at what you want to use them for, which herbs you are likely to use most frequently and what growing conditions you have. The following list gives suggestions of easy-to-grow herbs that are among the key herbs in the Herbal Detox Plan.

| Plant | Comments |
| --- | --- |
| Chamomile (*Matricaria recutita*) | Provides colour and scent. |
| Echinacea (*Echinacea purpurea*) | A stunning plant with pink to purple flowers; needs protection from slugs as a seedling. |
| Elecampane (*Inula hellenium*) | This is a tall herb with yellow flowers. It grows well against sunny walls. |
| Fennel (*Foeniculum vulgare*) | A vigorous plant with attractive foliage. |
| Figwort (*Scrophularia nodosa*) | Likes damp ground. |
| Garlic (*Allium sativum*) | Easy to grow from cloves, with attractive globe flower heads. |
| Globe artichoke (*Cynara scolymus*) | Grow as a vegetable; this tall plant has beautiful purple flower heads. |
| Golden rod (*Solidago virgaurea*) | Lovely small yellow flowers. |
| Marigold (*Calendula officinalis*) | Gorgeous orange flowers; will grow in vegetable beds or pots. |
| Marshmallow (*Althaea officinalis*) | Soft leaves and velvety flowers; likes to grow in damp, sunny places. |

| Plant | Comments |
|---|---|
| Milk thistle (*Silybum marianum*) | With its large thistle flowers and 'milk' splashed leaves this plant is always a talking point. |
| Nettles (*Urtica dioica*) | A patch of nettles will provide medicine, food (nettle soup), and attract useful insects to the garden. |
| Passionflower (*Passiflora incarnata*) | This climbing vine has remarkably complex and beautiful flowers and grows well on sunny walls. |
| Peppermint (*Mentha piperita*) | Grow in a bucket to prevent the roots spreading and taking over your garden! |
| Rosemary (*Rosmarinus officinalis*) | Likes a sunny spot. |
| Sage (*Salvia officinalis*) | Stunning foliage (red or green). |
| Skullcap (*Scutellaria lateriflora*) | Small herbaceous plant with pretty purple flowers, suitable for borders. |
| St John's wort (*Hypericum perforatum*) | Grows well in an open, sunny spot and provides beautiful flowers. |
| Thyme (*Thymus vulgaris*) | A low-growing plant; can be cultivated in pots or in cracks in paths. |
| Valerian (*Valeriana officinalis*) | Lovely clusters of pink flowers; likes soil to be damp. Grows well on stream banks. |
| Vervain (*Verbena officinalis*) | Provides marvellous delicate spikes of tiny pink flowers. |
| Yarrow (*Achillea millefolium*) | Grows easily, even on rough ground. |

Some herbs, such as lemon balm (*Melissa officinalis*) and many of the Mediterranean aromatic herbs, such as rosemary (*Rosmarinus officinalis*) like to be positioned in full sun on well-drained soil. Others, such as valerian (*Valeriana officinalis*) and meadowsweet (*Filpendula ulmaria*) appreciate partial shade and damp ground. If you are lucky enough to have some woodland or a woody area in your garden, you may be able to experiment with growing some of the forest species such as the North American golden seal (*Hydrastis canadensis*). Most herbs are resilient and pest resistant, and you should find it easy to grow them organically. Many are opportunistic, used to colonising whatever ground is available and do not require (or desire) the heavily fertilised soils often needed by vegetables.

One of the great things about growing herbs is that as well as getting wonderful food flavourings and remedies, you also benefit from the spin-offs, such as beautiful butterflies and useful insects coming into the garden, providing a delight to the eye and biological control for pests on your fruit and vegetables. You also get marvellous scent, colour, and leaf and flower variety.

## Harvesting

Different parts of herbs are harvested at different times. With pot-grown culinary herbs, just cut off what you need when you need it and leave the plant to replace what you have taken. Some medicinal herbs can be harvested more than once a year while others offer a single annual harvest.

When cropping medicinal herbs you should try and gather the herb when it is in its optimal therapeutic state. Generally, parts of the plant above ground should be harvested on fine clear days, ideally after one or two days without rain, during mid-morning or early afternoon when the dew has dried off and the sun is at its height. Never gather wet herbs for storing. Some people like to gather herbs in tune with the phases of the moon and stars. In general, one should harvest with the waxing moon as activity in plants appears to thrive during this period.

It is best to harvest a part of the plant before the next part of the plant develops. This means:

- **Roots** – gather while the plant is dormant in late autumn or very early spring before the above-ground parts of the plant regenerate.

- **Leaves** – gather when fully developed but before the flowers appear.

- **Flowers** – gather just as they open fully and before the fruits begin to appear.

- **Fruits and seeds** – gather just as they ripen and before they fall from the plant.

By gathering the parts at these times you are catching them while the plant is focusing on their development and concentrating energy into their tissues.

Biodynamic agriculture works very closely with the lunar calendar in terms of sowing and treating, as well as harvesting plants.

This advice on harvesting applies to both cultivated and wild plants, but there is a further point that needs to be made about wild plants. It is essential in the interests of plant conservation that you should only take locally abundant plants from the wild – and even then only very carefully. People have always harvested herbs and fruits from the countryside and this has tended to be a mutually beneficial and sustainable relationship. In more recent times with the mobility of communities and the encroachment of towns into the countryside, this relationship has lost its traditional safeguards. When harvesting from the wild, try to follow this code:

- Only harvest a plant when you are absolutely sure that you have identified it correctly. Failure to do so may result in gathering a toxic herb or in depleting a rare herb from the wild;

- Only harvest a plant when you find it in abundance. Do not take a single plant on its own or from a small group;

- When you do find an abundant patch of herbs, never take more than 10% of the supply;

- Avoid harvesting roots – if you only take above-ground parts then the plant has the chance to regenerate from its roots;

- If you do harvest roots, split the root, taking one half, and replanting the other so that it will re-grow.

## Storing

Once harvested, herbs need to be processed and stored for future use. The simplest and best way to prepare herbs for storage is to dry them.

- Spread out the herbs on plain paper on a kitchen table, sifting through and removing any diseased parts or any extraneous matter such as grasses, plants or soil. With roots, wash off any soil with cold water and gently pat them dry, then slice large roots into thin sections to speed up their drying time. Unsliced thick roots will take forever to dry and may rot in the centre.

- Leave the herbs to dry in a warm, dry, dark place – an airing cupboard or a place next to a central-heating boiler is ideal. Space the herbs out on paper, leaving gaps so that they are not overlapping. Leave for a few days, turning occasionally, until you can crumble the herb and it is completely dry.

Either store the herbs in brown paper bags or glass (ideally coloured brown, amber, green or blue glass as these prevent ultraviolet rays from the sun damaging the herbs). Never keep herbs in airtight plastic containers as any residual moisture will then be expressed and cause rotting. A good tip is to put the freshly dried herbs into a brown paper bag and then into a glass container so that the bag can soak up any remaining moisture – after a week or so remove the bag and discard it. Whatever you store your herbs in, keep them in a cool, dark place such as a kitchen cupboard away from sources of heat.

# Preparing and Taking Herbs

In order to promote optimum health it is useful to take herbal preparations that can be considered primarily as food products. There is a growing field of food products known as 'functional foods' or 'nutriceuticals'. These are foods with a specific nutrient or active herbal constituent content which have well-defined medical benefits. Traditional herbal preparations fitting this bill include:

- **Fresh or dried herbs** – used as flavourings in soups, stews, gravies and in vegetable, meat and fish dishes or combined with grains such as couscous.

- **Herb vinegars** – vinegars such as organic apple cider vinegar have cleansing and anti-inflammatory properties that are enhanced when combined with herbs. You can place a sprig of culinary herbs into good-quality vinegar and this will draw out and preserve its flavour as well as its therapeutic properties. Rosemary makes a really good herb vinegar.

- **Herb oils** – herbs can be infused in oils as well as vinegar and then used for salad dressings and for drizzling over dishes or using as an alternative to butter and margarine on bread. A wonderfully aromatic, tasty and invigorating herb oil can be made by infusing bruised basil leaves in olive oil – simply delightful!

There are many other types of herbal preparation. The ones referred to in this book and the ways in which they can be prepared and used are as follows:

## Teas

Taking herbs in tea form is perhaps the most effective way of using herbs on a day-to-day basis to improve general health.

Herbal teas can be made in two ways, by infusion or decoction. Infusions, sometimes called tisanes, are made by covering the herbs with hot water and leaving the mixture to brew before using, much in the same way as you would make a cup of China or Indian tea. This method is suitable for soft plant tissues such as leaves, flowers and fine seeds. Decoctions are made by simmering herbs in water in order to release the constituents contained within hard plant tissues such as roots, barks, waxy leaves, fruits and seeds. Before decocting hard plant parts, it helps to crush them in a pestle and mortar to make them easier to extract. Decoction is not recommended for plant parts that contain a lot of volatile oils as they can evaporate away during the process.

*To make an infusion*
Pour 250ml (a mug full) of just boiled water over 2–3 teaspoons of the herbs, cover over and leave to brew for 5 minutes, then stir, strain and drink. Take the tea 2–4 times a day.
You can brew herbs in a teapot or in a mug with a saucer over the top.

*To make a decoction*
Place 2–3 teaspoons of the herbs in a non-aluminium pan (stainless steel or enamel are ideal), pour on 300ml of water and simmer gently for 5–10 minutes. Then stir, strain and drink. Take the decoction 2–4 times a day.

To avoid having to make your infusion or decoction several times each day you can make up 2–4 cups at the same time, drink one cup and pour the rest into a thermos flask for use later in the day. This is especially useful when you are at work or on the move.

## Tinctures

Tinctures are liquid preparations of herbs in a water/alcohol mixture. They are very effective medicines but are more suited to the treatment of disease in professional practice than home use for the promotion of optimal health. The recommendation of this book is that for detox and general self-treatment with herbal remedies, teas are preferable to tinctures as they are gentler and more suited to everyday use.

## Creams and ointments

Ointments are fatty preparations that do not contain water and are poorly absorbed by the skin – they form a greasy layer over it. Creams are a mixture of water and fats and they form a soft layer that mixes with the skin and is absorbed into it.

Herbal creams and ointments are made with a suitable base cream or ointment preparation to which herbal preparations are added. Dried herbs are mixed with the base and melted together in a bain marie or slow cooker for around 2–3 hours, then strained. The liquefied, herb-infused base is left to set into a solid cream or ointment. Base materials can also have infused oils or tinctures added to them to make herbal creams.

If stored in a cool, dark place or in the fridge, creams will keep for 6 months to a year.

## Juices

Juices are made by pressing succulent fresh plant parts such as leaves, flowers, fruits and seeds. They should be drunk fresh unless a preservative is added. If you have a juicer, you can experiment with mixing herbs and fruits to make healthful drinks. Some commercial ranges of herb and vegetable juices are available.

Juices are particularly suitable preparations for use in detoxing since they are fresh liquids that are vibrant with enzymes and nourishing and cleansing constituents. Great detox juices include those of herbs such as nettle leaves, dandelion leaves, cleavers and chickweed. Carrot and radish juice is a good liver stimulant, beetroot helps to cleanse the lymphatic system, and garlic and onions can be added to juices to clear the lungs. Celery juice is good for the kidneys and urinary system. Herb and vegetable juices are generally more useful for detox than fruit juices as the latter are rich in sugars, especially when juiced and separated from their fibre content, which helps to prevent the sugar content from being released into the system too quickly when the fruit is eaten whole. An exception to this rule is lemon juice, which has excellent cleansing properties and is not too sweet.

## Infused oils

Infused oils are made by adding plant parts to a cold-pressed fixed oil such as almond oil, leaving the mixture to macerate and then straining the infused oil.

A hot infusion is used for extracting leaves – infuse the warmed oil and herb mixture in a bain marie (a glass bowl over a pan of simmering water will do fine) for 3–4 hours. A cold infusion is used for flowers – simply pour your fixed oil into a large glass jar full of the flowers until they are completely covered, then seal and leave to infuse for 2–4 weeks.

Once infused, strain the oil through a muslin bag and store in a dark-coloured bottle in a cool, dark place. The oil will keep for 6 months to a year. Infused oils can be added to creams and ointments or used as massage oils. Limeflower oil is wonderfully soothing and healing to dry or flaky skin.

## Tablets and capsules

Tablets and capsules are convenient ways to take herbal medicines, but they are not always as effective as liquid preparations such as teas and tinctures. They are made either from powdered dried herbs or from liquid preparations that have then been spray dried. It is often hard to get enough herbal content into tablets and capsules in terms of the volume of herbal material that is required to have a significant therapeutic effect. For this reason, high-potency tablets are generally to be preferred, although this does depend on the strength of the particular herb concerned. Having said this, do bear in mind the potential problems that high-strength standardised extracts may pose (*see* page 30).

## Compresses and poultices

Herbal compresses are formed by making a strong infusion or decoction of the required herb, soaking a cloth in the liquid, wringing it out and then applying the cloth to the affected area of the body.

A poultice is similar to a compress, but instead of applying an infusion or decoction of the herb to the skin you apply the herb itself. Poultices can be made with dried or fresh herbs and they are generally applied warm. Traditionally, a poultice of powdered slippery elm bark has been used as a drawing agent. It helps to soften and swell the skin, making it easier to extract foreign bodies such as thorns and splinters. It can also help to bring painful boils to a head.

Compresses and poultices are good ways of applying herbs to specific localised areas of the body.

## Gargles and mouthwashes

Gargles and mouthwashes are prepared from infusions, decoctions or tinctures. Prepare the required tea or dilute the tincture with water and use. For a gargle use a cup of tea or 5ml of tincture in a cup of water and gargle with sips of the liquid. Take a sip, gargle, spit the fluid out, then take another sip and repeat again. Continue to do this for about 5 minutes until the fluid has all been used. Use the same amounts of liquid for a mouthwash and swill sips of the fluid around the whole of the mouth, repeatedly flushing it around the tongue, teeth and gums.

## Baths

Herbal baths are made by adding infusions or decoctions to bath water, or by infusing sachets of herbs in the bath water itself. Use about 100g of herb for a full bath, with half that amount for foot or hand baths.

Foot baths are excellent at the end of a long day for easing tired feet, but they can also have more general effects. They are particularly useful for children who refuse to take herbs by mouth.

Hand baths can help to relieve the tension that can build up in the muscles of the hands, particularly in those of people using computers and factory machine operators who use their hands intensively for a living.

*Points to remember when taking herbal preparations*

- When taking herbs by mouth always ensure you dilute tinctures with water and wash tablets and capsules down with water. In order to minimise the chances of consuming pesticides and other potentially harmful chemicals, it is wise to use bottled mineral water or filtered tap water.

- If the herbs seem to hit you very quickly after taking them, or a little too strongly, or if they seem to be causing stomach irritation or indigestion, try taking them at the same time as food. This will slow down the absorption of the herbs.

- Taking herbs with food may be particularly useful in older patients.

- When applying herbs externally to the skin, always patch test a small area of skin first to see whether you have any intolerance of the particular plant being used.

# Chapter 4

# DEVELOPING YOUR HERBAL DETOX PLAN

The first three chapters have set the scene for the rest of the book. From this point you can begin to reflect on your own health and identify any areas that may need support or enhancement. By reading through the book, and making notes on the features that you feel apply to you, you will be able to draw up a personalised herbal detox plan.

The chapters in **Part II** explore basic herbal health concepts that can be used by everyone. These will form the foundation of your herbal health plan. They are:

- Detoxification (chapter 5),
- The use of herbal antioxidants (chapter 6),
- The use of herbal adaptogens (chapter 7).

It is a good policy for everybody to practise regular detoxification and consume a high level of antioxidants. Taking an appropriate adaptogenic herb gives a further dimension of health enhancement that complements these two strategies.

The chapters in **Part III** take a systems approach to the body, helping you to personalise your plan and focus on the elements relevant to you. Each chapter looks at a different body system:

- The immune system (chapter 8),
- The digestive system (chapter 9),
- The heart and circulation (chapter 10),

- The respiratory system (chapter 11),
- The bones, muscles and skin (chapter 12),
- The reproductive system (chapter 13),
- The mind and the emotions (chapter 14).

By reading these chapters you should be able to identify which (if any) tendencies, weaknesses or strengths you have in each area.

The major herbs that can be used to address your particular weaknesses or to promote optimum functioning are described, and for each system one key herb is described in detail; this herb is the single most useful and generally applicable herb for the system under discussion.

When taking herbs, remember that they can be slow and subtle in building up their effects, but once these accumulate they are deep acting and long lasting. To enable them to work best it is important to take them regularly and consistently. Taking a course of herbs is like reprogramming the body – herbs can change bodily habits and tendencies by correcting and expanding the activities of the body's organs, leading to improved general functioning.

By working with the programme described, you can expect to begin to reap the rewards of taking herbs for health in just six weeks. After this, using herbs will become part of your way of life.

*Caution*

This herbal health programme is not suitable for pregnant women, although it does present excellent strategies for couples wanting to improve their vitality and fertility before trying to conceive. Lactating women should discuss herbal treatment with a herbal practitioner before following any advice given in this book. Children's health can be enhanced with herbs, but parents or guardians should always first consult with a herbal practitioner to establish the best way to do this. One of the best ways of protecting your children's health and promoting their development is by adding antioxidant culinary herbs and foods to the diet (*see* chapter 6).

# The Outline Plan

The general plan covered here is simply a framework to point you in the right direction and get you started. You need to read the whole book in order to reap the full health-enhancing benefits of the herbal approach. In the outline plan below, you will be referred to relevant chapters for further details.

The plan is designed to promote exceptional health in people who are currently averagely healthy – if you are taking orthodox medication or have a significant medical condition you should consult with your doctor and a herbal practitioner before going any further.

A large number of herbs are mentioned in this book in order to offer you a wide range of potential herbal allies to select from. When reading through the book, take particular note of the descriptions of each herb in order to select those that seem to suit your own needs best. While most of the herbs mentioned are very easily obtained, some are a little obscure and you will need to contact a specialist supplier in order to obtain them. A list of such suppliers is provided at the end of the book (*see* Resources, page 268). The list below gives you a 'Starter's Pack' of ten of the most useful herbs that you will come across in the book and they should all be easily available. In addition, there are mentioned many important food herbs such as garlic, bilberries, ginger, rosemary, thyme and sage; these are widely available from food shops – or you can grow your own.

| Herb | Comments |
| --- | --- |
| **Dandelion** (*Taraxacum officinale*) This herb is a major detoxifying agent and is used for skin and digestive health. | Dandelion root is available in the form of 'Dandelion coffee'. Since this plant is so widespread you can also harvest the leaves and roots and dry them for your own use. |

| Herb | Comments |
| --- | --- |
| **Ginkgo** (*Ginkgo biloba*) An effective antioxidant; also improves circulation and memory. | Several gingko products are available from health food shops, including tablets and liquids. |
| **Siberian ginseng** (*Eleutherococcus senticosus*) One of the most broadly applicable adaptogens, used to improve mental and physical performance. | Many health food shops stock Siberian ginseng products and some have the dried root itself. Make sure you ask for Siberian ginseng, not Korean ginseng (*Panax ginseng*). |
| **Echinacea** (*Echinacea purpurea*) This is one of the best immune boosting herbs. | Many echinacea products are available, including capsules, tinctures and cough sweets. |
| **Chamomile** (*Matricaria recutita*) A calming and anti-inflammatory herb useful for soothing the digestive system, reducing headaches and aiding sleep. | Chamomile is one of the best-selling herbal teas and it is widely available in teabag form or as a loose dried herb. |
| **Hawthorn** (*Crataegus* species) The leaves, flowers and berries of this plant are protective for the heart and also have antioxidant properties. | Hawthorn teabags are available from health food shops. Some may also sell the loose dried leaves and flowers. |
| **Cloves** (*Syzygium aromaticum*) Cloves are warming to the circulation, help relieve colds and chest infections, and relax the digestion. | Dried cloves can be bought as a spice in food shops. |
| **Marigold** (*Calendula officinalis*) For improving skin tone and easing sore muscles and joints. It also stimulates immunity. | Marigold creams and tinctures are available from health food shops. The dried flowers are also readily available. It is also easily grown. |

| Herb | Comments |
|---|---|
| **Chasteberry** (*Vitex agnus-castus*) The key herb for correcting many of the problems of the female reproductive system. | Tablets and tinctures of this herb are available from health food shops. |
| **Valerian** (*Valeriana officinalis*) This is probably the most effective herb for protecting against the effects of stress. | Valerian preparations are available from most health food shops and pharmacies. |

You will find that Weeks 1 and 2 require the most effort on your part. After that it is just a question of making gradual refinements. It is imperative that you start the plan with a 'can do' attitude and use your willpower to make the initial changes, during which time you may not notice many benefits. The benefits *will* come but first you must make the necessary changes and persevere with them. The effects of herbal medicine accumulate gradually over a period of time – relax, be patient, and enjoy the vitality and energy that will come as you progress.

It is important to prepare the body for future improvements by clearing the way ahead with detoxification. Taking detox herbs is of limited value if the diet and home environment continue to be sources of congestion and pollution. The information below will help you to improve your diet and identify areas of your home environment where health-enhancing changes might be made.

# WEEK 1 – Dietary Changes and Detoxification

To begin the process of health transformation positively you need to start with a course of gentle detoxification, together with a reappraisal of your diet. (For more detailed information about detoxification, please read chapter 5.)

## Diet

The first thing you need to do is to identify and replace the foods that tend to cause congestion and damage to the body's tissues and cells.

Begin by making a list of the foods that you normally eat and drink throughout the day, as well as other substances that you take into your body, such as alcohol, tobacco and other drugs (prescription and otherwise). You may be consuming things that have no nutritive value and have only a negative impact on the body. Have a look at the list below and identify the items that you think you should reduce or cut out completely.

| Meals and other areas of consumption | Items consumed |
| --- | --- |
| Breakfast | |
| Morning snacks | |
| Lunch | |
| Afternoon snacks | |
| Evening meal | |
| Late snacks | |
| Fluids in the morning (e.g. tea, coffee, juices, water) | |
| Fluids in the afternoon (e.g. tea, coffee, juices, water) | |
| Fluids in the evening (e.g. tea, coffee, juices, water) | |
| Alcohol (units over the average week) | |
| Cigarettes | |
| Prescription drugs (from your doctor) | |
| Self-prescribed drugs (over-the-counter) | |
| Recreational drugs | |

You should now have a reasonable idea of the foods and other substances that you consume regularly. Now look at the list below, which identifies common problem foods and other substances that are detrimental to your health and makes suggestions on how to address these problems. This can involve reducing substances, replacing them or cutting them out altogether.

Be gentle on yourself and do not try to do too much at once. If the scale of the changes you need to make seems overwhelming do not despair – start by doing the things that you feel are either most important or most achievable and then gradually introduce further changes. You will find that as you start to feel better it will become easier to bring in further positive changes later on.

Some people may need specific diets – for instance if you suffer from or have a family history of sweet or fatty food cravings, obesity, late-onset diabetes or heart disease you should consider the Syndrome X Diet (*see* pages 253–7).

| Substance | Problem | Solution |
| --- | --- | --- |
| **Wheat** | Can cause food intolerances, bloating and lethargy. | It is important to eat a wide range of grains such as barley, rice, quinoa, millet and buckwheat – not just wheat. Buy a cookbook and learn how to prepare them. |
| **Dairy products** | Can cause mucus congestion and symptoms of intoler-ance. Cheese contains hard fat and this is one cause of arteriosclerosis (hardening of the arteries). | Do not eat dairy products excessively. Green vegetables, soya products, sardines, salmon, nuts, seeds, whole grains and pulses are alternative sources of calcium. |
| **Sugar and confectionery** | Cause tooth decay and are stored in the body as triglyceride fats, which contribute towards obesity, | Learn to take hot drinks without adding sugar or alternative sweeteners. Eat fruit as a substitute for confectionery. |

| Substance | Problem | Solution |
|---|---|---|
| | diabetes and heart disease. | |
| Cakes, pastries, biscuits, crisps, etc. | High in fat and/or sugar (*see* opposite). | Eat nuts and seeds as alternative snacks, and fruit salads as desserts. Try baked apples with dried fruit, rice or oat cakes with nut butters. |
| Fizzy drinks and squashes | High in sugar, artificial sweeteners and additives. May cause mood swings, hyperactivity, headaches and other symptoms. | Make water your main drink every day. If you need the fizz, try carbonated water with a twist of fresh lemon juice. |
| Fruit juices | High in sugar, low in fibre. | It is better to eat fruit than to drink fruit juices since juicing concentrates fruit sugars and removes the soluble fibre that is needed to prevent the sugars from turning to fat in the body. Substitute with blended whole fruit 'smoothies'. |
| Non-organic foods | May contain high levels of pesticides, herbicides and fertiliser residues. Non-organic meat may be high in antibiotics and growth hormones. | Try to eat as much organically grown food as possible. Try growing some of your own – if you do not have a garden you could rent an allotment. |

| Substance | Problem | Solution |
|-----------|---------|----------|
| Salt and high-salt foods | Can cause a rise in blood pressure in the 1/3 of the adult population who are 'salt-sensitive'. If there is a family history of high blood pressure this probably includes you. | Do not add salt to food and avoid processed products as these are often high in salt. Read labels and remember that salt is also called sodium and may be listed as this. |
| Tea and coffee | Tea contains tannins that can inhibit the absorption of vital nutrients, especially iron. Coffee is a stimulant that can cause anxiety and interfere with sugar metabolism and blood-pressure control. | Substitute with herbal teas such as chamomile, peppermint and lime-flower or rooibos (red bush) tea. Use barley/chicory-based substitutes for coffee. |
| Red meats | High in saturated fat and pro-inflammatory products (arachidonic acid). | Eat oily fish (such as tuna, sardines, herring, mackerel, salmon) and chicken in preference to red meat. |
| Saturated fat | Leads to a rise in cholesterol, heart disease and stroke. | Replace hard cooking fats (butter, margarine, animal fats) with poly- and mono-unsaturated fats such as olive oil. Avoid frying food: steam or grill it instead. Supplement the diet with a high-quality oil rich in omega 3 essential fatty acids such as hemp oil. |

| Substance | Problem | Solution |
|---|---|---|
| Alcohol | Can cause damage to vital body organs and lead to psychiatric disease if taken in excess. | Avoid binge drinking and drinking on an empty stomach. One or two glasses of red wine taken with meals may help to prevent heart disease. |
| Cigarettes | Cause cancer and contribute to the development of heart disease and strokes. | Should be avoided completely. Help may be needed to withdraw – herbal medicine and acupuncture may help. If you cannot cut them out then cut them down and take 500mg vitamin C daily, eat antioxidant foods (fruit and vegetables) and reduce your saturated fat intake. |
| Prescription drugs | May cause dependency and a range of side effects. | It may be very important to continue with your medication when the effects of stopping the drug are worse than the adverse effects it may cause. In some cases it may be possible to substitute with gentler natural therapies – always discuss this with your doctor and a qualified natural health care practitioner before making any changes. |
| Self-prescribed drugs | May cause dependency or side effects. | Some self-prescribed drugs may be of benefit but many |

| Substance | Problem | Solution |
|-----------|---------|----------|
| | | merely suppress symptoms (such as painkillers) or cause dependency (such as some laxatives). Your need for such drugs will decrease as your health improves. |
| **Recreational drugs** | May cause dependency and a range of side effects. | Although they may enhance creativity or a sense of well-being, they can also cause damage to the body and mind. Being optimally healthy provides a sustainable 'natural high' that many people find more satisfying than an artificially induced state. |

## Detoxification – level 1

The cleansing effect of rationalising the diet can be substantially enhanced by completing a course of herbal detoxification. There are several ways of working with detoxification and herbs, and these are covered in detail in Chapter 5.

A gentle but effective way of detoxing with herbs for Week 1 is to make a tea from a selection of dried herbs that work on improving the functions of the body's natural detoxification channels. A general detox tea for enhancing elimination via these routes could contain:

20g Burdock roots (*Arctium lappa*) for the bowels;
20g Dandelion roots (*Taraxacum officinale*) for the liver;
20g Celery seed (*Apium graveolens*) for the kidneys;
15g Yarrow leaves and flowers (*Achillea millefolium*) for the skin;
15g Thyme leaves (*Thymus vulgaris*) for the lungs;
10g Marigold (*Calendula officinalis*) for the lymphatics.

# WEEK 2 – Bringing In Antioxidants

By the end of Week 1 you will have cleared the way to make fundamental health improvements possible in the following weeks. Begin Week 2 by discontinuing the detox tea.

## Detoxification – level 2

In addition to detoxing the body with herbs and dietary changes, it is essential to lower the toxic load on the body by detoxifying your home environment. Below are the main things that cause pollution in the home and suggestions for what can be done about them. Much of this also applies to the work environment – if you can make these changes at work as well, then so much the better!

## Cosmetics, cleaning and decorating products

We use many chemical products in the home, including:

- **Cosmetics** such as shampoos, soap, make-up and perfumes;
- **Household cleaning products** such as washing powder, bleach, toilet cleaners and furniture polish;
- **Decorating products** such as paints and varnishes.

Many of these products contain noxious chemicals that deplete the immune system, causing allergic reactions and even cancer.

It is wise to avoid sprays including hairsprays and deodorants that can be inhaled and cause problems with the nose and lungs. Many waterproofing sprays and cat/dog flea sprays are highly carcinogenic – if you need to use them at all, use them out of doors and cover your mouth and nose.

Use products such as bleach sparingly, if at all – not only can they harm you, they can also harm the environment. There are many alternative products available which offer gentler options for ourselves and the planet. Products that contain artificial perfumes, colours and dyes tend to be highly aggressive substances that affect our health adversely and destroy animal and plant life. Choose unperfumed, biodegradable products. Organic paints are available that contain volatile oils from plants as alternatives to synthetic antifungal agents in conventional paints. In general, it is good to develop a questioning attitude towards everyday chemical products and ask, 'Is this safe? If not what is the healthy alternative?'

## Light pollution

It is natural for our bodies to spend time in both the light and the dark. In the daytime, it is important to be exposed to natural sunlight that our bodies need to produce vitamin D for the production of energy and the regulation of hormonal functions. The hormone melatonin – involved in promoting sound, healthy sleep and in repairing daily damage to the body cells – requires a dark environment to work effectively. In the daytime you should open the curtains and let light into the house; in the evening and at night it is better to use low-wattage energy-efficient lights, soft lamps and candles rather than bright bulbs and fluorescent strip lighting. At night you should sleep in the dark.

## Water pollution

Tap water can contain potentially harmful levels of chemicals, such as chlorine and fluoride, which are intentionally added to the water supply, as well as other non-intended constituents such as oestrogen and pharmaceutical drugs. Using a water filter, either plumbed in to your water supply or as a jug, can help to reduce the levels of many of these unwanted substances. Alternatively, you can use bottled water for drinking and save tap water for washing and cleaning.

## Atmospheric pollution

If you live in an area where the air quality is good, you should open windows and let fresh air into the house whenever possible. This will help to cleanse and refresh the atmosphere in the house and thus improve your energy levels.

A vacuum cleaner with an effective filter that traps dust and other allergenic particles will help you to remove these irritating substances from your home.

Being careful to regulate the temperature in your home is very important. Too much dry heat (such as from central heating) can dry the mucous membranes of the nose, throat and lungs, leading to an increase in respiratory infections, asthma and sore throats. If the home is too cold, this slows down the circulation and weakens the immune system. A damp atmosphere will also contribute to chest infections, fungal infections, and often exacerbates arthritis and rheumatism.

## Avoiding toxic furniture

Many new furnishings, including sofas and carpets, are coated with chemicals to make them flame retardant and resistant to fungal growth. Unfortunately, these chemicals can have harmful effects, including allergic reactions. When buying new furnishings it is a good idea to leave the windows open as much as possible in the room they are in and to avoid using that room for a few days while the excess chemicals disperse. Alternatively, you can choose natural products that are guaranteed not to contain chemical coatings.

## Tackling radiation

Whether or not electromagnetic radiation poses a significant threat to our health is still open to debate. There is enough evidence to make us cautious and some studies suggest that radiation may damage our immune systems and cause cancer. Although most attention has been on the problems associated with overhead electricity power lines, we should also reduce our exposure to low-frequency electro-magnetic field sources such as mobile phones, washing machines, microwaves, television sets and computers. Televisions and computers continue to emit electromagnetic fields even when switched off so it helps to unplug them from their sockets when not needed. In addition, sit as far back from them as possible when using them and keep the time spent using them to a minimum.

57

## Antioxidants

Chapter 6 is dedicated to examining this vital aspect of herbal healing, so please read through this chapter. Antioxidant plants (foods and herbal medicines) reduce the effects of the free radicals in your body which may cause damage to cell membranes and contents, potentially contributing to a number of disease processes, including the development of cancer and heart disease. Taking antioxidants regularly reduces the risk of these problems.

The major source of antioxidant supplementation is through the dietary intake of fruits and vegetables. From the beginning of Week 2, add to the dietary changes made in Week 1 by ensuring that you eat at least five servings of fruit or vegetables each day. Five should be an absolute minimum and a base line of ten a day would be better. This becomes easy if you can get into the habit of having raw fruit and vegetables as snacks in addition to cooked or raw vegetables with meals.

You should also give yourself an antioxidant boost from now until Week 6 by taking a herbal antioxidant and a nutritional antioxidant supplement to complement your fruit and vegetable consumption. A good antioxidant nutritional supplement will include vitamins A, C and E and the trace mineral selenium. Several herbs have strong antioxidant activity, so try to include the following in your meals: rosemary (*Rosmarinus officinalis*), turmeric (*Curcuma longa*), ginger (*Zingiber officinale*), and others listed in Chapter 6.

From Week 2 also take a tea made of either ginkgo leaves or hawthorn leaves and flowers (*Crataegus* species) each day to provide further antioxidant enhancement for your body.

# WEEK 3 – Adding Adaptogens

During Week 3, keep up the dietary changes you have made, and continue to work on eating plenty of antioxidant fruit and vegetables and improving your home environment. Continue with the nutritional antioxidant supplement and the herbal antioxidant tea.

The main addition for Week 3 is to introduce a herbal adaptogen into your health plan. For more about adaptogens, please read Chapter 7.

Adaptogens improve physical and mental performance particularly with regard to endurance and stamina. They help you to cope with the stresses of life in terms of physical and mental demands, and by means of their enhancement of immune functioning, they help to protect the body from the chemical stress of environmental pollution.

By reading Chapter 7 you should be able to decide which adaptogen is likely to suit you best. The most widely tolerated and effective adaptogen is Siberian ginseng (*Eleutherococcus senticosus*) and this will suit most people. Whichever adaptogen you decide to use, you can take it:

- As a tablet;
- As a liquid preparation (such as a herbal tincture);
- Or as a dried herb added to your antioxidant tea.

## WEEK 4 – Working with Your Herbal Allies

During Week 4, read carefully through Part III of this book and take notes about the herbs that seem to be appropriate for your health needs. These plants will become your personal herbal allies. Try to be selective and limit your choice to the two or three herbs that will be the most important for you.

Take these herbs in addition to the antioxidant and adaptogen herbs you are already taking. You may take them separately or combine them as dried herbs within a single tea mixture. It is easiest to combine the herbs to make a tea. At Week 4 you need to add 1–3 herbal allies to your 1 antioxidant herb and 1 adaptogen herb. This will give you a tea mixture with up to 5 herbs in it. Take the tea 3 times each day. Remember to take your herbs regularly otherwise they will not be able to accumulate their health-maximising effects.

# WEEK 5 – Helping the Herbs to Work

During Week 5 you should focus on your need for exercise and relaxation, and consider the ways in which you could meet these needs. Look also at the ways in which you can work with art and nature to improve your well-being. It is important that you reflect upon yourself as a whole individual and consider your needs as an emotional, mental and spiritual being as well as a physical one. Once you have decided on the things you would like to do, take positive action and make them happen. The information in each of the chapters in Part III will help you to decide which supplementary measures, beyond taking herbs, are right for you.

# WEEK 6: Review and Revise

As you enter Week 6 you will have:

- Revised your diet to engender health;
- Completed a week of detoxification of your body and started the process of detoxifying your home environment;
- Boosted the antioxidant activity in your body with food and herbs;
- Begun to harness the power of adaptogenic herbs to improve your strength, energy and immune resistance;
- Selected your herbal allies to address the areas of your health that need support;
- Begun to make changes in your lifestyle to fulfil your needs as a whole person.

By now you should be experiencing some definite improvements in your sense of well-being. These should be sufficient for you to feel that you want to carry on and optimise your health even further.

# After Week 6

- Discontinue the nutritional antioxidant supplement and the herbal antioxidant tea, but take them again if you ever feel in need of them.

- Maintain your intake of fruit and vegetables to sustain the beneficial changes to your diet.

- Continue to keep your home environment free from chemical, light and radiation pollution.

- Be prepared to take the herbal detoxification tea again, say for one week out of every six, if you feel the need of it.

- Continue with the adaptogen herb for another two weeks and following that take adaptogens on a regular basis. A general rule of thumb is to take adaptogens for six weeks and then to break for two weeks. Continue this cycle for as long as you feel that the herbs are helping.

- Change your herbal allies as the need arises. Some herbs (such as chamomile tea) may become part of your everyday diet, while others may only be needed occasionally.

Remember that working with herbs is a continuing process. The effects of following the simple but powerful strategies contained in this book can help protect you from developing major diseases. As the old saying has it, they will 'add years to your life and life to your years'. I hope you enjoy the experience.

See page 62 for an at-a-glance guide to the six week herbal detox plan.

Week 1    **Do:** Examine your diet and begin to make improve
         ments to it; read chapter 5 to help you to choose the
         detox herbs that are right for you.
         **Take:** Detoxification herbs.

Week 2    **Do:** Detox your living space; and read chapter 6 to
         help you select an antioxidant that suits you.
         **Take:** Antioxidant herbs.

Week 3    **Do:** Read chapter 7 to help you select an adaptogen.
         **Take:** Introduce an adaptogen herb, keep taking the
         antioxidants.

Week 4    **Do:** Read Part III to help you select your herbal allies.
         **Take:** Add up to 3 herbal allies to your adaptogen and
         antioxidants.

Week 5    **Do:** Use Part III to help you decide on any extra
         measures you can take to improve your health in
         addition to herbs; start to implement these.
         **Take:** Continue taking your herbal allies, adaptogen
         and antioxidants.

Week 6    **Do:** Continue to work on the extra measures you have
and       identified that you need. Continue with dietary
beyond    improvements and caring for your home environment.
         **Take:** The herbal allies, adaptogen and antioxidants
         until the end of week 6. Continue to use detox,
         antioxidant and adaptogen herbs from time to time
         and to bring in new herbal allies as they are needed.
         *Keep coming back to the book for advice whenever your
         health needs support.*

# PART II

# Weeks 1–3

The three steps covered in the first three weeks of the Herbal Detox Plan are:

- **Week 1** – Cleanse the body;
- **Week 2** – Protect the body;
- **Week 3** – Improve the body's performance.

The initial detoxification work will help to cleanse your body and set the scene so that the transformation of your health can begin. Adding in antioxidants will start the process of enhancing your health by providing protection against damage by diet, environmental pollution and the ageing process. Bringing in an adaptogen will help you take the first steps towards improving the way your body functions and this will lead to improved energy levels and a greater sense of well-being.

## Week 1

Chapter 5 looks at the crucial role that detoxification can play in cleansing and revitalising the body and it covers the most useful herbs that can be taken to achieve effective detoxification. In Week 1, you should examine your diet and modify it to reduce the burden on the detoxifying organs and to help keep your body clear of potentially harmful dietary factors (see Chapter 4). In addition, you will select the herbs that seem best suited to your detox needs (or follow one of the general-purpose mixes recommended) and take a detox tea throughout the first week.

## Week 2

Chapter 6 explores how you can benefit from taking an optimum intake of antioxidant containing foods and herbs. In Week 2, you will discontinue the detoxification herbs and replace them with an antioxidant tea or supplement. The information in Chapter 6 will help you to choose the antioxidant herbs that will best meet your needs. In Week 2, you will also extend your detoxification work from your body to your environment, making sure that your home and work environments are as free of harmful influences as possible (see Chapter 4 for more on this).

## Week 3

Chapter 7 describes how adaptogens can improve your mental and physical stamina and endurance, and help to protect you against the effects of stress. It goes on to detail the uses of the adaptogen herbs and helps you to select the herbs that are likely to work for you. During Week 3, you will also continue to take the antioxidant herbs that you chose in Week 2.

# Chapter 5

# DETOXIFICATION –

## Herbs for rejuvenation and renewal

Detoxification is one of the central healing concepts in herbalism. A course of herbal treatment may often begin with a preparatory period of detoxification to clear the way for more specific treatment. But detoxification also has an essential role to play in normal daily life as a strategy for promoting optimum health. Periodic detoxification will help to cleanse and revitalise your body, helping it to function more efficiently and making you feel better.

Detoxification has grown in popular understanding to have certain links, particularly in connection with fasting, colonic irrigation and as a part of treatment for cancer.

### Fasting

Although detoxification is often associated with fasting, in fact fasting is instinctive and appropriate during acute infections. When fasting, the body does not need to expend energy on digesting and assimilating food and can instead mobilise its forces to attack the invading infection. Short fasts of 24–48 hours can also be of great benefit for some medical conditions and can promote general well-being. Herbal detoxification can be combined with fasting for occasional deep cleansing or with a more pure diet for more regular cleansing.

## Colonic irrigation

The use of enemas has played a role in various forms of medicine for many years, including herbal medicine, although their use is not so frequent today. Proponents of the Gerson therapy, developed by Max Gerson as a form of cancer treatment, sometimes use coffee enemas to stimulate the liver as part of a detoxification programme. Colonic irrigation may be indicated in the treatment of certain conditions but I do not generally recommend it.

## Cancer treatment

Detoxification is a traditional herbal approach to treating tumours. Tumours were seen as areas of congestion or blockage that needed 'opening up' with eliminative herbs in order to clear the channels and let the vital force flow freely again. Over recent years, Essiac, a traditional Native Canadian herbal formula, has attained a wide reputation as a possible cancer treatment. I would not suggest that Essiac is a panacea for cancer – quite clearly it is not – but this and other herbal detoxification treatments may have a supporting role to play in the treatment of some cancers.

In the context of this book, what is more important is that regular detoxification may have a role to play in preventing some cancers appearing in the first place. A regular cleansing routine may help to prevent the accumulation of carcinogenic substances within the body, thereby reducing our 'toxic load' to levels that our body can easily process, thus preventing any impairment of our health.

# About Toxins

There is a strong modern interest (some might say an obsession) with detoxification nowadays. This is perhaps understandable when we consider the levels of pollution in the world today. Patients and practitioners both talk about wanting to cleanse the body of toxins, but what exactly do we mean by this?

Toxins are substances that damage or impair natural bodily functions; specifically they are agents that have negative effects on cellular structure or function. They can be produced within the body (endogenous toxins) or come from outside (exogenous toxins). Toxins include:

- **Heavy metals** – such as lead, mercury and aluminium. These derive largely from environmental pollution by the manufacturing industries and by motor vehicles. We may also come into contact with them through daily activities such as cooking (with aluminium pans and utensils), eating food from tin cans (which may be soldered with lead compounds), having mercury amalgam fillings in our teeth, and using certain paints and cosmetics.

  Heavy metals can cause vague general symptoms such as headaches and fatigue. They can also cause cancers and some studies have shown an association with neurological disorders such as attention deficit hyperactivity disorder (ADHD) in children and Alzheimer's disease in the elderly.

- **Harmful chemicals** – such as solvents, preservatives (like formaldehyde), agrochemicals (pesticides, herbicides, growth promoters), medical drugs (including vaccines), recreational drugs (including alcohol and tobacco) and food additives. Of particular concern here is that some products we use around the home daily (such as cleaning agents), foods that we eat regularly (particularly processed foods and non-organically grown foods), and medical drugs all have the potential to cause toxic damage to our bodies. While herbal detoxification can be beneficial in offsetting this problem, it should be noted that many herbs, including several that are not widely considered to have marked detoxifying properties (such as St John's wort – *Hypericum perforatum*), improve the liver's ability to process and eliminate toxins from the body. Conventional therapeutic drugs are largely metabolised in the liver and so herbal stimulation of detoxification by the liver may result in impairing the effectiveness of a drug. If you are taking prescribed medication, you should talk to your doctor and your herbalist before beginning a programme of herbal detoxification.

- **Microbial compounds** – as the body processes the breakdown products of micro-organisms such as bacteria and yeasts, some of their toxic constituents can accumulate and cause damage to healthy cells. Toxic microbial debris in the bloodstream may lead to the development of allergic and autoimmune diseases. Autoimmune diseases are those where the body attacks itself. They may arise because our immune systems react against a compound made up of normal body cells attached to microbial toxins. Efficient removal of the products of microbial degeneration from the body using herbal detoxification may help to prevent such diseases developing.

- **Metabolic residues** – if the normal products of bodily metabolism are allowed to accumulate they can cause damage to cells and trigger inflammation. Elements such as the breakdown products of body proteins can cause particular problems. Improvement of liver and kidney functioning with herbs can reduce this problem.

Looking beyond these groups of toxic agents, it is relevant to consider how we might respond to the issue of environmental toxicity and see how it relates to the emotional, mental and spiritual levels of our being.

## Environmental toxins

We need to consider environmental detoxification alongside personal detoxification because our own health and the health of the world are intimately linked. Pollution may be airborne (industrial and vehicular toxins), carried in the water (industrial chemicals), or held in the soil (agrochemicals). As well as this, there is the greenhouse effect, caused by the burning of fossil fuels, and the thinning of the ozone layer caused by the action of the sun on the pollutant CFCs.

Clearly, the solution to many of these toxic problems can only come from large-scale political initiatives. As individuals, though, we are not powerless. We can campaign for political change and we can work as individuals, families or groups to look at issues such as our own energy consumption and production, car use, and our repair, reuse and recycling habits so that we may help to effect change from the ground up. Our major tool is our buying power – if we refuse to buy polluting goods and non-organic foods, then we will help to cut back their production.

## Mental toxins

You may also have a desire to work with spiritual as well as physical detoxification – cleansing the emotions and mind of negative responses, patterns and thoughts. Many of us feel congested and overloaded psychically as well as physically and this is understandable since we are exposed to excessive quantities of information, images and sounds. Much of this could be termed mentally toxic.

In a religious or mystic sense, physical cleansing has long been associated with spiritual purification. We tend to have negative images of this tradition, visualising religious fanatics denying themselves the pleasures of life and punishing their bodies to 'free the soul'. While this has been the case, purification need not be puritanical; it should not be about denial and suppression but about balance and liberation. Herbal medicine is a holistic outlook and although we are largely focusing here on herbal detoxification at a physical level, it is worth complementing this by also considering how we can be careful about what we put into our hearts and minds as well as into our mouths.

# Herbal Detoxification

## An Evolving Art

Detoxification has long been a mainstay of the herbalist's craft but the approach has evolved over time. Traditionally, herbal detoxification used very strong herbs to effect an extreme cleansing of the body. Detoxification was seen as particularly important because it was a tangible way of working with the four humours and their corresponding four fluids – phlegm, blood, black bile and yellow bile. Herbs that caused vomiting or violent evacuations of the bowel gave potent evidence of successful manipulation of the body's essential fluids! Detoxifying herbs are classed in categories such as the emetics (causing vomiting), purgatives and cathartics (causing pronounced bowel movements). Such measures may have been useful in treating poisonings (including food poisoning) if caught at an early stage; the emetic herb ipecac (*Cephaelis ipecacaunha*) is still used in conventional medicine in cases of drug or chemical poisoning.

Such extreme measures are now rarely called upon and are not relevant here. Modern herbal medicine focuses on working with the body's channels of elimination in a gentler way, although strong laxatives are still indicated in some people with severe constipation. The emphasis is on promoting optimum functioning of eliminative processes and clearing toxins from the body, thereby helping to establish a clear flow of energy through the body.

At one time, many of the herbs used in detoxification were described as blood cleansers or blood purifiers. While it is true that the blood is a major channel for the movement of substances around the body, the main targets for detoxifying herbs are the organs the blood interacts with.

## Herbs for detoxification

The main eliminative channels in the body are in the:

- Bowel,
- Liver,

- Kidneys,
- Skin,
- Lungs,
- Lymphatic system.

Although the lymphatic system is not strictly a major eliminative channel, I have included it in this list because it plays an important supporting role in detoxification.

## Bowel

The prime function of the bowel (small and large intestines) is to absorb nutrients from the food we eat and to eliminate waste matter from the body. If bowel movements are reduced, then both absorption and elimination may be impaired. Herbs that stimulate bowel movements and that are suitable for general detoxifying purposes include:

- Burdock root (*Arctium lappa*);
- Yellow dock root (*Rumex crispus*);
- Figwort root (*Scrophularia nodosa*);
- English and black walnut, husks or inner bark (*Juglans regia* and *Juglans nigra*).

If you tend towards pronounced constipation, stronger bowel herbs may be needed (*see* page 138). If you have irritable bowel syndrome (IBS) or tend towards having very loose motions then these herbs should be avoided.

## Liver and gall bladder

The liver is one of the most important detoxifying organs and one of the most important organs in herbal medicine. There are numerous herbs that influence its functions. The liver produces bile which is stored in and released from the gall bladder. Bile itself has mild laxative effects on the bowel, and several herbs act on the liver, gall bladder and bowel together.

The liver is the prime site of detoxification for many drugs (medical and otherwise) and other toxic chemicals. It also processes many of the body's hormones, especially the steroidal hormones such as oestrogen. The liver is also crucial in the metabolism of carbohydrates, fats and proteins.

Key herbs stimulating liver and gall bladder detoxification include:

- Dandelion root (*Taraxacum officinale*);
- Oregon grape root (*Mahonia aquifolium*);
- Fumitory leaves (*Fumaria officinalis*);
- Chinese magnolia vine fruits (Wu Wei Zi – *Schisandra chinensis*).

Several herbs have a protective effect on the liver and are particularly useful for those whose livers may be at particular risk from chemical damage, for instance for those people whose occupations bring them into regular contact with petrochemicals. These herbs will also help protect us during periods of excessive alcohol intake. (This is not an excuse for heavy drinking or an insurance policy against damage; they will not protect the liver from the effects of sustained heavy drinking). Liver-protecting herbs include:

- Globe artichoke leaves and root (*Cynara scolymus*);
- Milk thistle seed (*Silybum marianum*);
- Hare's ear root (Chai Hu – *Bupleurum falcatum*).

### Kidneys

Although the liver is widely recognised as a detoxifying organ, the kidneys are sometimes overlooked. In fact, the liver and kidneys are close partners in detoxification, both having vital roles to play. Any well-rounded detoxification formula will work on both organs. As well as being responsible for controlling the concentrations of constituents in the body's fluids, it is in the kidneys that most of the waste products of the body's metabolism are excreted.

Many of the herbs that stimulate kidney functions are diuretics, improving the formation and excretion of urine. Most herbal diuretics are very mild and this is a good thing since overstimulation of urine production can deplete the body of vital elements and unbalance the body fluids.

Herbal kidney stimulants include:

- Golden rod leaves and flowers (*Solidago virgaurea*);
- Celery seed (*Apium graveolens*);
- Birch leaf (*Betula* species);
- Dandelion leaf (*Taraxacum officinale*);
- Couch grass roots (*Elymus repens*);
- Corn silk styles and stigmas – these are the long threads, which are the female parts, lying under the husk and covering over the meal of sweet corn or maize (*Zea mays*).

Several herbs have a reputation for protecting the kidneys from damage, improving their integrity and ensuring optimal functioning. These include:

- Parsley piert leaves (*Aphanes arvensis*);
- Pellitory-of-the-wall leaves (*Parietaria judaica*).

### Skin

The skin has the capacity to remove toxic products from the body through perspiration. This is one of the principles behind the use of saunas. In Native American sweat lodges, water was poured onto hot stones in the centre of a small circular tent where participants would gather to be purified by the steam. Sweat lodge ceremonies were often used as places for cleansing and meditative preparation before sacred rituals. After coming out of the lodge it was common to bathe in a nearby river to wash away the sweat and exuded waste products.

A group of herbs known as diaphoretics have the ability to induce perspiration. The perspiration triggered is usually mild, though still valuable. Diaphoretics work much more strongly when taken during an acute fever or during a sauna or sweat lodge session.

Herbal detoxification diaphoretics include:

- Elderflowers (*Sambucus nigra*);
- Limeflowers (*Tilia* species);
- Yarrow leaves and flowers (*Achillea millefolium*);
- Boneset leaves (*Eupatorium perfoliatum*).

*Caution*

Because diaphoretics improve blood flow to the skin, they can sometimes exacerbate some skin conditions, particularly eczema. Use with care if you have a sensitive skin problem.

## Lungs

The whole of the respiratory system from the nose to the smallest bronchiole in the lungs is lubricated and protected by a layer of mucus. The mucous membranes lining the respiratory system contain fine hairs called cilia, and these propel the mucus towards the top of the trachea (windpipe). From there, mucus is either swallowed or coughed up. The mucus also traps and removes inhaled pollutants from the body. Optimal performance of this 'mucociliary' lining is vital for protecting the body from exposure to external toxins.

Herbs stimulating the mucociliary system are known as expectorants. These loosen dried and thickened mucus and enhance the movement of the cilia. Expectorants are particularly useful for those who work in a polluted city environment or who regularly encounter an environment with dust or fumes. While it is better not to smoke at all, if you are a smoker then regular consumption of expectorant herbs is advised.

Effective herbal expectorants include:

- Thyme leaves and flowers (*Thymus vulgaris*);
- Elecampane roots (*Inula hellenium*);

- Hyssop leaves (*Hyssopus officinalis*);
- White horehound leaves (*Marrubium vulgare*);
- Fennel seeds (*Foeniculum vulgare*);
- Angelica seeds (*Angelica archangelica*);
- Gumplant leaves and flowers (*Grindelia camporum*).

### Lymphatic system

The lymphatic system is a major component of the immune system, as well as providing a series of drainage channels to allow excess bodily fluids in the spaces between body cells to empty into the veins. This drainage function is very important in supporting the efficient removal of waste products and toxins from the body. Lymphatic herbs can help ease congestion in the eliminative channels of the body.

Important lymphatic stimulant herbs include:

- Cleavers leaves and stems (*Galium aparine*);
- Sweet violet leaves (*Viola odorata*);
- Marigold flowers (*Calendula officinalis*);
- Echinacea roots (*Echinacea purpurea*).

## Benefiting from herbal detoxification

In the traditional understanding, detoxification removes blockages within the body, allowing the vital force to move through the body unimpeded. In a modern sense we can say that by improving the performance of the main detoxifying organs, we enhance their ability to keep us free from the harmful effects of toxins and waste products. A decongested body becomes capable of responding more quickly and emphatically to the demands placed upon it. Clearing the detoxifying organs helps to improve the general circulation and releases energy that is normally wasted on coping with the body's toxic load. In practical terms this results in better energy levels, enhanced resistance to disease and a greater sense of well-being. Regular detoxification may also help reduce the risk of developing serious diseases such as cancer and autoimmune conditions.

Detoxification may be particularly useful if you suffer from any of the following conditions:

- Fatigue,
- Catarrhal congestion,
- Chronic sinusitis,
- Otitis media,
- Skin diseases,
- Allergies,
- Food intolerances,
- Arthritis.

Regular detoxification is recommended for people living or working in polluted environments such as inner cities, near main roads or in congested offices, as well as for those people whose occupations put them particularly at risk by working with toxic substances.

*Cautions*
There are a few reasons to be cautious with detoxification and it is as well to be aware of these:

- Detoxification should normally be avoided during pregnancy and lactation; these are times for nourishing and building up the body rather than cleansing and clearing the systems.
- Avoid detoxification if you have a serious medical condition unless upon the advice and under the supervision of an experienced healthcare professional.
- Be cautious if you are taking medication from your doctor.
- If you are fasting while undertaking a herbal detox, do not prolong your fast for more than 24–48 hours, unless upon the advice and under the supervision of an experienced healthcare professional.
- Detoxification can lead to a sudden release of toxins within the system causing a mild shock to the system. As stored

toxins circulate, they may cause disruption until they are cleared from the system. Symptoms of detoxification can include: headaches, skin rashes, nausea, fatigue, irritability, altered bowel habit, flatulence and indigestion. These symptoms should ease and disappear after a short time. If symptoms persist or are severe, consult your healthcare practitioner.

Side effects are more likely to be experienced in individuals carrying a larger toxic load. As a rule of thumb, the more congested and toxic you think you are, the gentler you should be initially in your detoxification regime.

## Detoxing

There are several ways that herbs can be used to assist cleansing and renewing the body, either on their own or in conjunction with specific practices such as fasting. Deep herbal detoxification is best carried out under the advice and supervision of a herbal practitioner.

## Teas

Teas are by far the best sort of preparation for detoxing with herbs; the purifying effects of the plants are enhanced by the high water content and the absence of any other additives.

### General detox tea

A useful general detox tea, combining herbs from each of the categories listed above, would contain:

20g yellow dock roots (for the bowels)
20g oregon grape roots (for the liver)
20g birch leaves (for the kidneys)
10g elderflowers (for the skin)
20g elecampane roots (for the lungs)
10g cleavers leaves and stems (for the lymphatic system)

This mix adds up to 100g and it will provide treatment for about a week. You will see that higher amounts tend to be given for roots –

this is because roots and seeds give less volume of active ingredients for their weight. Generally, it is necessary to prescribe root and seed doses at twice those of other parts. The tea should be made by decoction (*see* page 39) at a dose of 2 teaspoons of the mix per cup. It can be taken at an intake of 3–4 cups a day for Week 1 of the Herbal Detox Plan.

For a deeper treatment, take the above tea in conjunction with a 24–48 hour fast. Take 4–6 cups of the tea in each 24-hour period and additionally drink at least 1–2 litres of water per day. You can also take vegetable juices such as carrot and beetroot in addition to the herbal tea. If you want to follow a herbal fast such as this it is best to do it over a weekend or on days when you are not working, so that you can spend time resting and sleeping rather than exerting yourself.

## Protective tea

For people working in polluted environments such as pubs, clubs, inner city offices, factories and for those working with toxic substances such as paints and solvents, this tea will help detoxify and protect the liver, kidneys and lymphatic system. It is gentle enough to use continuously over a long period of time. It would be best to take it during the working week and then take a break from it on your days off.

50g milk thistle seeds (for the liver)
25g parsley piert leaves (for the kidneys)
25g cleavers leaves and stems (for the lymphatic system)

100g will provide treatment for 1–2 weeks. The tea should also be made up as a decoction (*see* page 39), and it helps if you can pulverise the milk thistle seeds in a pestle and mortar before making it up. Use 2 teaspoons to a cup and take the tea 2–3 times a day.

## Everyday teas

There are several herbal teas that are readily available in teabag form and provide an easy way of integrating detox support into your day-to-day diet. Simple teas suitable for regular daily use include:

- Peppermint,

- Elderflower,

- Fennel,

- Nettle,

- Dandelion leaves,

- Dandelion root coffee.

Try to choose organically grown teas that have nothing added to them. Check the label to make sure that the tea does not contain any added colours, flavourings, sugar or caffeine.

## Diet and lifestyle

In addition to taking herbal teas, an ongoing detox approach should include modifications to diet and lifestyle. These are dealt with in some detail in Week 1. In a nutshell, this means trying to eat pure foods and accessing pure environments as frequently as possible.

In terms of purifying the diet:

- Avoid highly processed or refined foods;

- Make a habit of reading packets, looking at the ingredients lists and rejecting unsuitable products;

- Replace the beverages in your diet with single herb teas as mentioned above;

- During warm weather eat plenty of raw vegetables as salads and in colder weather eat plenty of root vegetable soups and greens;

- Try to eat organic produce whenever possible;

- Start and end your day with a mug of hot water – that's it, nothing added. It is amazing how cleansed this can make you feel;

- Make sure you drink 1–2 litres of water per day to help dilute toxins and wash them out of the body;

- Designate one day a week when you only eat raw foods and drink herbal teas – it does not have to be the same day each week.

In terms of getting in touch with pure environments, this obviously depends on your living circumstances but try and 'get away from it all' as often as possible and spend time in clean places such as hilltops and mountains and by lakes and seas. If it suits you, then hill walking and walking coastal paths can provide excellent exercise combined with lungfuls of revitalising pure air!

## KEY HERB FOR DETOXIFICATION

## DANDELION

**Scientific name** *Taraxacum officinale*

**Plant family** Asteraceae (Daisy family)

**Type of plant** Perennial herb.

**Parts used** Roots and leaves.

**Phytochemicals** Vitamins and minerals (A, B, C, D, potassium and calcium); sesquiterpene lactones; triterpenes; phenolic acids; polysaccharides; carotenoids.

**Actions** Aperient (roots); bitter tonic; cholagogue; detoxifying; diuretic (leaves).

**Indications**
**Roots** Liver disorders, arthritis, skin diseases, constipation, gallstones.
**Leaves** High blood pressure, oedema (swelling) associated with heart failure, gallstones.

**Preparations**
**Roots** Decoction.
**Leaves** Infusion; or eat fresh as salad leaves.

**Combinations** Dandelion roots and leaves combine perfectly with each other in teas. Traditionally, dandelion and burdock (*Arctium lappa*) were mixed together as a spring cleansing tonic drink. Dandelion leaves combine well with nettles in teas and soups.

**Cautions** Avoid dandelion root if you suffer from irritable bowel syndrome or have a tendency to loose bowels; only use on professional advice if you are taking significant conventional medication. Avoid dandelion leaf if you are taking a conventional diuretic drug ('water tablet') unless on professional advice.

**Conservation** Dandelions are widespread and generally considered as weeds.

# Chapter 6

# HERBAL ANTIOXIDANTS –

## Feeling better, living longer

One of the most important discoveries in medicine in the twentieth century was the understanding of the role that antioxidant compounds play in our health. Antioxidants help prevent cellular damage and degeneration, as well as having the potential to reduce the risk of cancers and heart disease. We can work with antioxidants, integrating them into our daily lives through diet and herbal supplements, so promoting optimum health and improving our well-being in our later years.

Antioxidants are substances that are used to target the metabolic products in the body called free radicals. Free radicals are produced as part of our normal bodily processes, and several of them serve useful and important functions – for instance, they are thought to play roles in growth, and in defensive and memory functions. Unfortunately, free radicals also have a negative side and their levels in the body need to be kept in check.

As well as being generated as a result of normal processes, free radicals are produced in large quantities in chronic infectious and inflammatory disease; they are also created in response to environmental toxins (such as air pollution, agrochemicals, food additives, cigarette smoke, conventional drugs, radiation and excessive exposure to sunlight). They are unstable molecules that react with cells, oxidising them and so causing damage to the cell membranes and the cellular contents (proteins and DNA). Antioxidants neutralise free radicals, thereby protecting cells from the destructive effects of oxidisation.

Free radical damage is associated with a wide range of diseases including autoimmune disorders (such as rheumatoid arthritis) and neurological conditions such as Parkinson's disease. Most significantly, it is associated with the development of the two main causes of death in the West – cancer and heart disease. It is also probably one of the main mechanisms behind the process of ageing itself.

Damage to DNA by free radicals can lead to gene mutations that initiate cancer. Further free radical attack can foster the progression of cancer. In heart disease, the major problem with free radicals is their impact on fats in the body. When levels of antioxidants are low, LDL cholesterol ('bad cholesterol') is more likely to become oxidised; when oxidised this fat sticks to artery walls more readily and this leads to hardening of the arteries (arteriosclerosis).

With regard to ageing, it is suggested that the continuing free radical damage over a period of many years leads to the development of errors in cellular DNA. This means that the body gradually loses the ability to regenerate itself. It has been estimated that the DNA in every cell in our bodies is exposed to oxidative damage by free radicals up to 10,000 times every day. Most of these attacks are immediately repaired, but the body relies on an adequate antioxidant intake from the diet to support the repair mechanisms. Antioxidant supplementation from herbs and the diet is the key to minimising this risk.

## Using Antioxidants

All the conditions below may benefit from optimum antioxidant intake:

- **Cancer** – prevention of some types;
- **Heart and vascular disease** – coronary artery disease, stroke, varicose veins, capillary fragility;

- **Disorders associated with ageing** – glaucoma, cataracts, macular degeneration, osteoarthritis, senile dementia and Alzheimer's disease;
- **Autoimmune disease** – rheumatoid arthritis, inflammatory bowel disease (Crohn's disease and ulcerative colitis);
- **Neurological disease** – Parkinson's disease, multiple sclerosis;
- **Liver disease**;
- **Allergic and hypersensitivity diseases** – asthma;
- **Male infertility**.

Among the diseases associated with ageing, macular degeneration stands out as the most common cause of visual impairment in older people in the West. Antioxidant intake seems to be very effective in decreasing the risk of visual problems as we age. But antioxidants have effects beyond the prevention of terminal and late onset illness.

- Free radicals are produced in greatly enhanced numbers during inflammatory disease such as inflammatory bowel disease. Antioxidant treatment may quell symptoms and reduce disease progression by enhancing free radical neutralisation and limiting further damage, thus helping to break the vicious cycle of disease progression.
- Antioxidants have an impact on *Helicobacter pylori*, the bacteria that causes stomach ulcers.
- Their role in the prevention of liver disease is largely achieved by inhibiting the build up of harmful fats in the liver.
- High levels of free radicals are found in the sperm of 40% of infertile men leading to deformation of the sperm produced. Antioxidant intake may be both preventative and curative here, with vitamin E being an especially important antioxidant in this case.

For all these conditions, it is very much the case that prevention is better than cure. Generally, these are areas where, once the condition is established, a cure is difficult if not impossible. While antioxidant therapy may alleviate some symptoms and help to slow the progression of these disorders, its real value lies in inhibiting their development in the first place. Of course, these conditions tend to have more than one cause, but the neutralisation of free radical damage by optimum antioxidant intake can still lessen their severity or even prevent them entirely.

Lastly, achieving optimum levels of antioxidants may lead to increased longevity but, more importantly, antioxidants could help us to be healthier during our whole lives, and particularly in our final years, where we can enjoy the fruits of experience in good health rather than struggling with significant chronic disease. While ageing is a natural process, it need not necessarily be a painful and disabling one.

## Types of Antioxidant

Antioxidants are found in plant foods and medicinal herbs. We can divide plant antioxidants into two basic groups, the nutrient antioxidants and the non-nutrient antioxidants. Major nutrient antioxidants include:

- Beta-carotene (provitamin A),
- Vitamin C,
- Vitamin E,
- Selenium.

The main non-nutrient antioxidants are the flavonoids and tannins. Both nutrient and non-nutrient antioxidants can be found in plant foods, but medicinal herbs mostly contain non-nutrient antioxidants.

### Non-nutrient antioxidants
#### Flavonoids
One of the major classes of antioxidants is the flavonoid group. This is subdivided into three categories:

- Flavones,
- Flavonols,
- Flavonones.

Flavonoids are pigment compounds that give colour to flowers and fruits. They are found in many plants especially herbs, fruits and vegetables. The word 'flavonoid' is derived from the Latin word *flavus*, meaning yellow, and many flavonoid-rich plants are yellow or orange in colour. The most important flavonoid compounds possessing potent antioxidant activity include quercetin, kaempferol and apigenin.

### Tannins

The tannins are a group of plant antioxidants closely related to the flavonoids. There are several types of tannins and some are used in herbal medicine for their ability to bind proteins together, causing an 'astringent' effect on tissues. This is useful in wound healing and treating diarrhoea. Antioxidant tannins include the proantho-cyanidins (or oligomeric procyanidins – OPCs). Two products rich in OPCs have been developed from grape seed (*Vitis vinifera*) extract and maritime pine (*Pinus pinaster*) extract. A related group of antioxidants, the anthocyanins, gives the red, blue and purple colours to fruits and flowers.

The flavonoids and tannins account for most of the antioxidant activity of medicinal herbs and they are also found in foods.

## Nutrient antioxidants

The nutrient antioxidants work together synergistically – each enhances the functions of the others. For instance, there is a particularly close relationship between beta-carotene (which is the precursor of vitamin A), vitamins C and E, and selenium. For beta-carotene to convert to vitamin A it requires vitamin E; the transportation and storage of vitamin E requires selenium; and vitamin C is responsible for regenerating vitamin E. Taking a supplement containing all of these ingredients will provide strong antioxidant support.

# Benefiting from Antioxidants

To gain full benefit from antioxidant foods, you will need to develop a dietary regime that optimises your intake of antioxidants.

## Food and drink

Most people are aware of the advice to eat at least five servings of fruit and vegetables combined each day. The aim of this is to boost our antioxidant levels and help prevent heart disease and cancer. In fact, the original research advised that we consume at least ten servings each day but government health bodies decided that a target of five a day would be more realistic. As it is, only 10–20% of people in the West are though to meet this reduced target. For anyone who does find this difficult, it would be wise to take a daily antioxidant nutritional supplement (*see* page 89). This should not be considered as a replacement for fruit and vegetables, but as a complement. Nutritional supplements are often poorly absorbed and can never be a total substitute for eating whole foods.

The following general advice will help you to achieve optimum antioxidant nutrition:

- Eat plenty of fruit and vegetables. Yellow, orange, red, blue and purple fruit and vegetables tend to be high in antioxidants, but do not neglect to eat greens.

- Antioxidant fruit and vegetables include:

| | |
|---|---|
| apples | grapefruit |
| apricots | lemons |
| aubergines | onions |
| beetroot | oranges |
| blackcurrants | peppers (red, orange, yellow, green) |
| carrots | pumpkin |
| cherries | quince |
| chillies | spinach |
| bilberries | strawberries |
| blueberries | sweet potatoes |
| grapes (red, black) | tomatoes |

- Eat a wide variety of fruit and vegetables.

- Eat fruit raw and eat vegetables raw as well as cooked.

- Eat the peel or skin of fruit and vegetables whenever possible.

- Choose organically grown produce as much as possible.

- Favour fresh foods over frozen and avoid canned products.

- Eating whole fruit and vegetables is better than taking juices.

- It is important to eat whole grains, nuts and seeds to gain antioxidant minerals and trace elements – eat a variety of grains such as barley, millet and quinoa, not just wheat; useful seeds include pumpkin, sesame and sunflower; useful nuts include almonds, Brazils, cashews and walnuts.

- Soya beans contain important antioxidants such as isoflavones and phenolic acids – incorporate soya products such as tofu and tempeh into your diet.

- Olives are rich in antioxidant flavonoids and tannins.

## Alcoholic drinks

The relatively low levels of coronary artery disease in the French population (by Western standards) may be due to its consumption of antioxidant compounds (tannins and other polyphenols) found in red wine. The French have a diet that is high in fat but it seems that this may be offset to some degree by the consumption of red wine. Research shows that the antioxidant activity of alcoholic drinks is not limited to red wine – whisky (specifically single-malt whisky greater than 12 years old), cider and some beers contain potent antioxidant polyphenols. (Please do not get carried away – alcohol can cause severe problems, including liver disease and psychiatric disorders.) The beneficial effects on the heart of some alcoholic drinks, particularly red wine, can be helped by following these guidelines:

- Only drink with meals, never on an empty stomach;

- Drink small amounts regularly (up to 2–3 glasses of red wine daily) rather than large amounts irregularly; binge drinking is particularly harmful;
- For every glass drunk take an equal volume of water;
- Have 1–2 days a week that are entirely alcohol free.

## Supplements

It is useful to take a broad-based antioxidant supplement to help ensure that optimum antioxidant targets are being met. A well-rounded supplement should contain the following substances at around the daily intake levels (for a healthy adult) suggested:

| | |
|---|---|
| Vitamin C | 250–500mg |
| Vitamin E | 100–200mg |
| Beta-carotene | 10–15mg |
| L-cysteine | 0.5–1.0g |
| Coenzyme Q10 | 30–100mg |
| Selenium | 50–100µg |
| Zinc | 15mg |
| Manganese | 5.0–7.5mg |

# Herbal Antioxidants

For convenience, I have divided the types of herbal antioxidant into those that are mainly used for culinary purposes, those that can be considered as safe daily beverages for continual use, and those that should be seen more specifically as truly medicinal herbs and should therefore be used with more caution. In practice, many of the herbal antioxidants that you take will fall into more than one of these categories.

## Culinary herbs

Many of the culinary herbs have antioxidant properties, often because they contain an antioxidant compound called rosmarinic acid. The regular use of culinary herbs in your diet is an easy way of enhancing the antioxidant properties of your meals. You can use fresh or dried herbs in soups, stews, vinaigrettes, sauces, gravies, and in vegetable, meat and fish dishes. Try growing herbs in pots in a sunny kitchen or on a window sill – you can immediately spice up a sandwich with a sprig of fresh basil or some finely chopped thyme.

First-class culinary antioxidant herbs include:

| | |
|---|---|
| Basil | Oregano |
| Cloves | Rosemary |
| Cumin | Sage |
| Garlic | Thyme |
| Ginger | Turmeric |

Curry spices tend to be highly antioxidant and it is a good thing to eat curries regularly. Turmeric, in particular, is a strong antioxidant with anti-inflammatory properties; research has shown that it may have a vital role to play in reducing the risk of developing Alzheimer's disease.

## Dietary herbs

There are a few herbs with strong antioxidant qualities that are particularly well suited to being taken on a regular basis. Such herbs can be used as substitutes for tea and coffee as daily beverages.

Since I am suggesting replacing 'ordinary' tea, a mention should be made of its healthier alter ego, green tea. Green tea and black ('ordinary') tea are made from exactly the same plant – the tea shrub *Camellia sinensis*. Black China or India tea is made from leaves that have been left to oxidise as they dry, turning black in the process. This oxidisation process removes most of the antioxidant polyphenols from the tea. By contrast, green tea is made by lightly steaming the fresh leaves to retain their green colour and halt the process of oxidisation, thus preserving the polyphenol content. This means that green tea offers a much more actively antioxidant alternative to black tea. In order to maximise the benefits of green tea, take it just as it is, infused in hot water without adding any milk or sugar.

There is a downside to green tea in that it contains caffeine and other stimulant substances called theobromine and theophylline. Some people may find these stimulants uncomfortable and so they should avoid green tea.

My favourite antioxidant herbal beverage, which has the benefit of being both a potent antioxidant and caffeine free, is made from the leaves of a South African shrub. Its botanical name is *Aspalanthus linearis* and it is known commonly as rooibos (or rooibosch), which is Afrikaans for 'red bush' as the leaves and the resulting tea made from them have a reddish-brown tinge. Rooibos is a popular alternative to black tea and coffee, with a very pleasant and distinctive taste and aroma, much gentler than black tea. It may take a week or so to get used to, but even hardened tea addicts have said that they much prefer it and will never take black tea again.

Thyme, as well as being a culinary herb, makes a very aromatic beverage – it is an acquired taste but, if the taste suits you, it can provide an excellent, very strong antioxidant for regular use as a tea.

## Medicinal herbs

Many herbs have strong antioxidant properties. My favourite, most commonly used medicinal antioxidants are the following:

**Hawthorn** (*Crataegus* species) – hawthorn leaves, flowers and berries are all used in herbal medicine. For antioxidant support it is best to take the leaves and flowers combined as a tea – this can be made by infusion at a dose of 2 teaspoons to a cup with 3–4 cups drunk each day. Hawthorn contains oligomeric procyanidins (OCPs) and it is particularly beneficial if you suffer from angina, high blood pressure or heart disease, or if there is a family history of these conditions. This is an especially good antioxidant for men who, through lifestyle and family history, may be particularly at risk of heart disease. If you suffer from low blood pressure or if you have been prescribed drugs by your doctor to lower your blood pressure, you should only take hawthorn on professional advice; otherwise, this is a very safe and widely tolerated herb.

**Ginkgo** (*Ginkgo biloba*) – the leaves of the ginkgo tree contain antioxidant flavonoids and they can be taken as an antioxidant tea by most people. However, for those taking conventional anticoagulant or antiplatelet drugs such as warfarin, it should only be taken on professional advice. Gingko is especially suited to older people.

**Meadowsweet** (*Filipendula ulmaria*) – the leaves and flowers of meadowsweet have good antioxidant properties and can be taken as a pleasant aromatic tea that also has anti-inflammatory and digestive properties. It can be taken as a regular tea and is especially useful if you tend towards joint, muscle or digestive problems such as indigestion or heartburn.

Other antioxidant herbs include:

Allspice fruits (*Pimenta dioica*)
Boldo leaves (*Peumus boldus*)
Chiretta leaves (*Andrographis paniculata*)
Dan Shen root (*Salvia miltiorrhiza*)
Ginger roots (*Zingiber officinale*)
Globe artichoke leaves and roots (*Cynara scolymus*)
Grape seed extract (*Vitis vinifera*)
He Shou Wu roots (*Polygonum multiflorum*)
Horse chestnut seeds (*Aesculus hippocastanum*)
Liquorice roots (*Glycyrrhiza glabra*)
Maritime pine (*Pinus pinaster*)
Milk thistle seeds (*Silybum marianum*)
Milk vetch root (*Astragalus membranaceus*)
Spruce needles (*Picea abies*)
Willow bark (*Salix* species)
Witch hazel (*Hamamelis virginiana*)

## Herbal cosmetics

Some herbs have antioxidant effects that can be used in cosmetic products. This is an area of herbal therapeutics that is growing rapidly at present. Horse chestnut seeds (conkers) have been used in leg creams to treat varicose veins, and witch hazel leaves (which contain antioxidant tannins) have been used to make an 'anti-ageing' face cream that inhibits wrinkle formation.

### KEY HERB FOR USE AS AN ANTIOXIDANT

## BILBERRY

**Scientific name** *Vaccinium myrtillus*

**Plant family** Ericaceae (Heather family)

**Type of plant** Deciduous shrub.

**Part used** Fruits.

**Phytochemicals** Anthocyanins; condensed tannins; oligomeric procyanidins (OCPs); flavonoids; phenolic acids.

**Actions** Antioxidant, anti-inflammatory, astringent, vasoprotective.

**Indications** Glaucoma; haemorrhoids; Raynaud's syndrome; retinal bleeding; retinitis and as a general antioxidant.

**Preparations** Fresh fruit eaten; decoction of dried fruit; bilberry jam. The fluid extract of bilberries made at a strength of 1:1 (where 1ml of the liquid preparation = 1g of dried bilberry fruits) is the antioxidant supplement that I most often prescribe, taken at a dosage of 3–6ml per day for adults.

**Combinations** Best taken by itself.

**Cautions**  Patients with bleeding disorders or taking anticoagulant or antiplatelet drugs ('blood thinners') such as warfarin should only take bilberry on professional advice.

**Conservation**  Bilberry is common throughout most of its range and is widely cultivated.

# Chapter 7

# HERBAL ADAPTOGENS –

## The key to enhanced performance

Adaptogens are compounds that improve vital capacities such as immune resistance and enhance physical and mental performance, helping to establish greater levels of endurance and stamina, and increased powers of concentration and memory. They help us to cope with the pressures of modern life, supporting the body and mind in dealing with the effects of stress. They also generate feelings of greater vitality as they help the body adapt to external and internal influences, so that it is better able to resist the development of fatigue, depletion and disease. They nurture the vital force throughout the body, strengthening it and improving its general resilience. They improve immune function, promote cell growth and longevity, support adrenal gland functions (particularly the production of the natural anti-stress hormone cortisol), improve liver functioning, and strengthen the nervous system.

The group of chemical constituents that are common to most of the adaptogen herbs are the triterpenoid saponins. These are complex, sugar-based chemicals with remarkable properties; other adaptogens are based on sugar molecules called polysaccharides – as a result, most adaptogens taste sweet. In the terms of Chinese medicine, these sweet-tasting plants are known as 'harmony herbs'. This is an appropriate phrase since harmony is the state that these herbs foster in the body – a state of balance, poise and resilience. However, this needs to be qualified because, in fact, most adaptogens taste bitter-sweet – there is an equal tone of bitterness combined with the saccharine taste. This is a further reflection of the chemical balance within the adaptogen herbs, bitter is the opposite of sweet and the one complements the other. We tend to love the sweet taste of things and generally dislike bitter-tasting foods. Consequently, we tend to suffer from an excess of sweetness leading to obesity, diabetes and heart problems. Adaptogens provide the feelings of satisfaction and completion associated with sweetness, but balance these with the grounding and enervating effects that bitters have on the body.

Adaptogens restore vitality in weakened, depleted and fatigued people, increase feelings of energy, and enhance our resistance to disease. They have also been shown to protect against radiation damage (this may help people who work with computers); they improve our mental capacities, enhancing our learning, and tend to improve libido and sexual performance. When described like this, adaptogens sound almost too good to be true but they really can offer huge benefits in terms of optimising our vital functions. They are the genuine life-enhancing feel-good herbs.

## Using Adaptogens

Adaptogens are the ideal herbs to support us in the stressful modern world and can be used by most adults. In particular, you should consider taking adaptogens if any of the following descriptions applies.

- You are an athlete.
- You work in stressful conditions.
- You regularly travel long distances (especially if you do a lot of driving or long-haul flying).
- You have to work to pressurised deadlines or work unsociable hours (particularly night workers).
- You feel fatigued, below par, tired and exhausted, or you suffer from recurrent minor infections such as coughs and colds.

- You have young children – adaptogens can really help you to cope, particularly in the demanding first 2–3 years following the birth.

Traditionally, adaptogens were taken more by older people in order to bolster deteriorating natural capacities and to shore up physical and mental reserves. Nowadays, many younger people need the support that adaptogens offer and will benefit from the protective effects that they provide against cancer and heart disease. I tend not to advise adaptogens for children since it is better to draw out and develop the innate vital energies that children possess – a healthy child should not need adaptogens.

It may appear that there are few of us who would not benefit from adaptogen supplementation, but not all adaptogens will suit everyone and they can lead to overstimulation. In particular, *Panax ginseng* should be avoided by people who are highly stressed and hyper-active. If you are overactive and hyped up you do not need ginseng but rather the herbs that will relax and nourish the nervous system described in Chapter 14. Adaptogens are there to help us cope with the demands of modern life but they should not be used as a prop to attempt to support an unsustainable lifestyle. Many of us need rest and recuperation, not rocket fuel! If you are highly stressed it is important to look beyond adaptogens to your diet, lifestyle, relaxation activities and attitudes towards work, relationships and 'life, the universe and everything'.

*Caution*

Despite the fact that adaptogens improve immune-system functions, they should not be taken during acute infections. The traditional view is that when someone is in an acute infective state, adaptogens are likely to 'strengthen the pathogen' rather than the person. However, they are suitable for aiding recovery from infection and should be taken during the convalescent period, not at the height of infection – when there is fever, diarrhoea or vomiting, and a need to stay at home or in bed.

## Ginseng

Ginseng is the most famous adaptogen, but the name 'ginseng' has come to be used for several different plants. When we think of ginseng it is most likely to be Korean or Asiatic ginseng (*Panax ginseng*). This is the best-known type of ginseng, although it is not the most suitable for many people.

Korean ginseng is a member of the Araliaceae plant family (the ivy family) which also includes two other very important ginsengs: Siberian ginseng (*Eleutherococcus senticosus*) and Canadian or American ginseng (*Panax quinquefolius*). These two are generally more suited to contemporary Western life and I use them more frequently than Korean ginseng in my practice.

It is difficult to classify the ginsengs in terms of their adaptogenic strength, but in terms of their stimulating quality, Korean ginseng is probably the strongest, followed by Canadian ginseng, with Siberian ginseng the mildest. Strongest does not necessarily mean best, however, and Siberian ginseng is the most commonly used in my practice, followed by American ginseng, with Korean ginseng only being used occasionally. The therapeutic reason for this is that Siberian ginseng is the best tolerated and most widely applicable type of ginseng, with the others being less so. There is another important reason though.

From a conservation standpoint, both Korean and Canadian ginseng are listed as endangered species by the Convention on International Trade in Endangered Species (CITES), so it is important that we consume these herbs carefully and only use guaranteed sustainably grown products. Korean ginseng is widely farmed, while Canadian ginseng is cultivated to a lesser extent, so it is possible to obtain ethical preparations of these plants.

Although Korean ginseng is a mighty herb, providing powerful healing benefits in some conditions, it has qualities that can make some conditions and situations worse. Korean ginseng should not be taken if you have high blood pressure or if you suffer from anxiety, acute asthma attacks, heavy periods or heavy nosebleeds. It should not be taken in conjunction with other stimulants (drugs or caffeine) or if you are taking blood-thinning drugs such as warfarin.

Liquorice (*Glycyrrhiza glabra*) is often taken alongside adaptogens as a complementary herb to improve their effects. Although moderate liquorice consumption is not a problem it can be a potential danger if you have high blood pressure – people with this condition should completely avoid preparations offering a combination of Korean ginseng and liquorice.

Although Siberian ginseng is gentler and safer than Korean ginseng, it remains an extremely effective adaptogen capable of fostering profound improvements in health. This makes it the best type of ginseng for general use.

There are a number of myths and confusions about ginseng. One of these is that Korean ginseng is the best type of ginseng for women and Siberian ginseng is the best type for men, or even vice-versa, but this is inaccurate and misleading. Both types of ginseng can be used by both sexes in appropriate circumstances. A number of plants are known as 'ginsengs' even though they do not belong to the ginseng family (Araliaceae). Although they have taken on the name 'ginseng' on account of their supposed wide-ranging powers, some are adaptogens but others are not. The most commonly encountered 'false ginsengs' are:

- **Women's ginseng** (or female ginseng) – this is a title sometimes given to Dong quai (*Angelica sinensis*) which is a member of the celery family (Apiaceae). It is not an adaptogen although it does have a wide range of uses in conditions of the female reproductive system.

- **Brazilian ginseng** – this term is sometimes used to describe the South American vine, guarana (*Paullinia cupana*) which is a member of the Sapindaceae family, a group of tropical trees, shrubs and climbers. It is not an adaptogen (although it has been marketed along these lines) because although it contains saponins, its main stimulant activity is based on a chemical group called xanthines, which includes caffeine, theobromine and theophylline.

- **Indian ginseng** – this is a term occasionally applied to
  ashwagandha (*Withania somnifera*), a member of the potato
  family (Solanaceae). This *is* an adaptogen and is profiled
  below.

## Tonics and adaptogens

Most of us are familiar with the idea of 'taking a tonic' and probably
consider a tonic to be something that 'builds you up', 'gives you
energy' or 'keeps you going'. These phrases all describe activities of
the adaptogens.

Tonics improve the 'tone' and therefore the performance of the
body's organs but they are not necessarily adaptogens. In herbal
medicine, there are tonics that support and enhance the functions of
particular parts of the body, such as the heart, or liver or kidneys. These
tonics are rarely adaptogens in the true sense, although some are, such
as the liver tonic Chinese magnolia vine (*Schisandra chinensis*).

There is a long history of tonic drinks, the most famous of all
being Coca-Cola. This was originally based on the leaves of the coca
shrub (*Erythroxylum coca* – the source of cocaine) and cola nuts (*Cola
nitida* – a high caffeine source) and was used by frontiers people
developing homesteads in the American west. Another was sarsa-
parilla (*Smilax* species), which was popular for building up muscles
and energy. Most of our modern tonic drinks are based on caffeine
and/or glucose, and give a short burst of energy followed by a reflex
depletion of energy. These cannot be considered in any way healthy
and they are the very antithesis of adaptogens.

## The Major Adaptogenic Herbs

The adaptogen herbs are a small and elite group. Below you will find
profiles of some of the most widely used and important members of this
group, together with a couple of lesser known 'up and coming'
contenders. In Russia, where much of the research into adaptogens has
been carried out, it is common practice to cycle the intake of adapto-

genic herbs, typically taking them for six-week periods separated by two weeks off. This is good advice when using adaptogens for general health promotion as it provides a regular 'washout' period, thus preventing the body from becoming over reliant on the herbs.

Preparations and dosages for the individual herbs are described below. Do note the cautions listed throughout this section.

## Korean ginseng (Asiatic ginseng)

The botanical name of this plant is *Panax ginseng*. This is the best-known type of ginseng but it is not always the best suited for general use. The name 'Panax' derives from the Greek word *panacea*, meaning 'cure all', giving us an indication of its strong therapeutic reputation. This herb has most of the attributes of adaptogens and has been used to treat a wide variety of conditions, but its major claim to fame has been its reputed ability to enhance longevity. It is mainly considered as an adaptogen for the elderly rather than for younger people because its stimulatory effects can prove excessive. It can be beneficial in promoting the levels of HDL cholesterol ('good' cholesterol) thereby reducing the risk of heart disease, in reducing the risk of some cancers, and in treating impotence and fertility problems in men (another reason for its high demand, having long been considered a 'herbal viagra'). It can be of benefit to individuals with alcohol and drug dependency who are trying to conquer their addictions and return to good health. The dosage for healthy adults is 0.5–3.0g per day of the dried root by decoction or 1–6ml per day of the tincture (at a strength of 1:2), but do note the cautions to the use of this herb discussed on page 98 and bear in mind its conservation status.

## American ginseng (Canadian ginseng)

American ginseng (*Panax quinquefolius*), although overshadowed by its more famous Asian relative *Panax ginseng*, is a very important type of ginseng. Traditionally, it was used by Native American tribes for a host of problems: the Cherokee used it for headaches, coughs, colic, 'nervous affections' and as a tonic; the Creeks took it for skin problems, colds and shortness of breath; the Iroquois used it for tapeworm, ear aches, sore eyes, fever and tuberculosis; and several tribes employed it as a general tonic or panacea. The Chinese imported American ginseng in large quantities, firstly from Canada then later from America. A number of Canadians and Americans became 'seng diggers' to meet the Chinese demand. Surprisingly, most of the writers from the Physiomedicalist and Eclectic herbal approaches writing around the late nineteenth and early twentieth centuries consider American ginseng to be a minor remedy – perhaps it lacked the forcefulness that many of the severe conditions affecting people at those times required. Today it fits a niche by providing a remedy similar in effects to *Panax ginseng*, but it is better tolerated and less aggressively stimulating. This form of ginseng tends to be better suited to Westerners than Korean ginseng although it is now endangered in the wild. Only supplies of the root that are certified as being ethically sourced should be used. The dosage for healthy adults is 1–4g per day of the dried root by decoction or drunk as a powder or 2–8ml per day of the tincture (at a strength of 1:2).

## Siberian ginseng

Siberian ginseng (*Eleutherococcus senticosus*) is probably the best adaptogen for general use because it is both gentle and effective, lacking the problems associated with *Panax ginseng*. Also, it is not an endangered species and it is much easier to obtain high-quality supplies of the herb and at a better price. For these reasons, Siberian ginseng is the key herb for this section and a detailed profile is given at the end of the chapter. It grows through eastern Russia to Korea, China and Japan. The best example I have ever seen was growing in a herb garden on the Black Isle near Inverness in Scotland. Russian research has

developed the profile of this herb and extensive studies of its
effectiveness were carried out on factory workers and truck
drivers. These studies showed that workers taking Siberian
ginseng were less likely to take time off due to illness. In the
1970s and early 1980s, the plant was taken by Russian
cosmonauts and by athletes preparing for the Olympic Games.

## Milk vetch root (astragalus, Huang Qi)

The botanical name for this herb is *Astragalus membranaceus* and
it tends to be referred to as astragalus rather than by its common
names. It is a perennial herb originating in Asia and has long
been used as a tonic in traditional Chinese medicine. It is
primarily used as a well-tolerated stimulant to the immune system
and has even been used as a supplementary treatment for cancer.
It is useful for chronic viral infections, especially *Herpes simplex*.
Traditionally, it has been used as a tonic to the blood and was
taken following blood loss. It is a useful adaptogen for women
who have a tendency towards heavy bleeding during their
periods. An important attribute of this plant is that it helps to
lower blood pressure and this makes it an ideal adaptogen if you
suffer from hypertension or heart disease. Astragalus is taken
either as a decoction of the whole dried root or by consuming the
finely powdered root – in each case the dose used for healthy
adults is 2–6g per day. Alternatively, you can take the tincture (at
a strength of 1:2) at a dosage of 4–12ml per day. Astragalus is
considered to be a very safe herb and suitable for general use.

## Chinese magnolia vine (Wu Wei Zi)

The fruits of *Schisandra chinensis* are an important remedy in
traditional Chinese medicine, where they are used to treat coughs,
insomnia and impaired memory. Recent research has shown that
they have protective effects on the liver. They have a role to play
in cancer prevention and improving physical endurance and

mental performance. Studies have demonstrated an enhancement of eyesight and hearing when taking this herb. It may therefore be a very useful adaptogen for use if you have liver problems or are experiencing deterioration of your vision or hearing. It should be avoided in pregnancy, except on professional advice. The dosage is 1.5–6g per day of the dried fruit by decoction or 3–12g of the tincture (at a strength of 1:2) for a healthy adult.

## Gotu cola (gotu kola)

The newer botanical name for this plant is *Centella asiatica* but you may find it still referred to by its older name of *Hydrocotyle asiatica*. Gotu cola is a trailing herbaceous plant, sometimes called Indian pennywort, that grows in India and Pakistan, where it is used in salads or eaten as a vegetable. It also grows from China to Australia, as well as in parts of Africa. It has become popular in herbal practice as a herb to help with the healing of wounds, due to its pronounced influence on tissue regeneration. It has been used for treating burns, cellulite, varicose veins and varicose ulcers, post-operative scars, acne scars and wounds, and has long been used for treating a vast range of skin problems in Ayurvedic medicine.

Beyond this, gotu cola has several adaptogenic properties, including a traditional reputation for enhancing longevity and a proven capacity to improve mental performance. It was one of the constituents of a formula used by the Chinese herbalist Li Ching Yun, who died in 1933 at the (reputed) age of 256! Gotu cola helps to relive anxiety and the effects of stress, and it has been used for infertility, insomnia, tiredness, depression, memory loss and sexual fatigue.

It is perhaps best regarded as a mild adaptogen that may be of particular benefit if you have arthritis, skin problems or problems with concentration or memory. The leaves are taken as an infusion at a dosage of 2–4g per day or as a tincture (at a strength of 1:2) at 4–8ml per day. This plant is considered to be safe and well tolerated but it should not be confused with cola (*Cola nitida*), which is simply a stimulant containing caffeine and is in no way an adaptogen. The related European marsh pennywort (*Hydrocotyle vulgaris*) is not currently used by herbalists but was mentioned by Culpeper as a treatment for kidney stones.

## Ashwagandha (winter cherry)

*Withania somnifera* is a fascinating herb. It grows from Africa to India and has long been used in Ayurvedic medicine as a tonic and aphrodisiac, to improve learning and memory functions, and to treat a wide range of conditions including asthma, skin diseases and insomnia. It has been used as an aid in preparing racehorses and the common name 'ashwagandha' means 'strength of a horse'. This plant has the full range of adaptogenic attributes – it has antitumour properties, enhances physical and mental performance, and protects against the effects of ageing. But it has a further property, quite rare amongst adaptogens, in that it has a calming and relaxing effect on the body in addition to enhancing energy levels. It therefore may be very suitable if you suffer from anxiety or overactivity and are worried about the stimulant effects of many adaptogens. In my own practice, I have found it to be useful in cases of depression especially in men. It is certainly useful for male impotence where the cause is exhaustion and fatigue. The dosage is 3–6g per day of the root by decoction or 6–12ml per day of the tincture (at strength of 1:2) for a healthy adult.

## Reishi mushroom

Herbal medicine uses all types of botanical substances including fungi. Fungi differ from green plants in that they do not produce chlorophyll, but they do produce several substances that can improve our health. The reishi mushroom (*Ganoderma lucidum*) contains triterpenes called ganoderic acids and polysaccharides (chains of sugar molecules) that boost the immune system and have anticancer properties. Reishi is a bracket fungus that grows like a small shelf on trees, particularly oak trees, and on old tree stumps. This type of mushroom is as hard as wood. It is scarce in the wild and is largely cultivated. In China it is known as 'the mushroom of immortality' due to its association with increased longevity. It is used in herbal medicine for high blood pressure, chronic fatigue syndrome, the neuralgia that follows *Herpes zoster* infection (shingles), and as a treatment for cancer and HIV/AIDS. Japanese research has shown that reishi inhibits the development of the virus that causes AIDS, but more research is needed to demonstrate how useful taking the mushroom might be in treating the condition. Alongside *Panax ginseng*, the reishi mushroom is one of the most widely used and highly esteemed adaptogens in China. Large-scale cultivation means that it is now more widely available. The dosage is 1–2g of the dried fungus per day, prepared as a decoction or taken in tablet form.

## Rose root (golden root, arctic root)

Rose root (*Rhodiola rosea*) is currently receiving interest as a new adaptogen. In fact, it has been used in Russia for many years and researched over the last 30 years. It certainly shows a lot of promise as a major addition to the ranks of adaptogens. It is a member of the Crassulaceae family, which includes the stonecrops (*Sedum* species) and houseleeks (*Sempervivum* species). It grows in mountainous and arctic areas of Europe and Asia, including sea cliffs in Western Scotland and Ireland.

Traditionally it has been used to treat depression and high-altitude sickness, to improve general mental and physical performance, and to relieve states of fatigue. Research shows that it has protective effects on the heart and against cancer. It may be particularly suitable if you suffer from high blood pressure, insomnia or chronic fatigue syndrome. Like ashwagandha, it appears to have antidepressant and calming effects as well as improving energy levels.

Perhaps the most interesting thing about rose root is that it seems to act quickly whereas most adaptogens build up their effects gradually. This means that it could be useful for treating acute episodes of stress as well as chronic ones. If you suddenly find that your stress levels have increased dramatically for whatever reason, then rose root may be one of the best adaptogens to take to achieve a rapid increase in support for the body.

One of the main active constituents is a glycoside (sugar molecule) known as salidroside or rhodioloside, but it is clear that the chemistry of this plant is complex. Studies using the standardised extract at high doses have shown contradictory activity, including some cases of blood pressure increase and insomnia. My advice would be to avoid the standardised extract and use the whole natural root instead. Take a decoction of the root at a dose of 3–6g per day or the tincture (at a strength of 1:2) at a dosage of 6–12ml per day, for a healthy adult.

## Devil's club

The wonderfully named devil's club has an equally lovely botanical name – *Oplopanax horridus*. The 'horrid devil's club' reference comes from the fact that this shrub is extremely thorny and can be vicious if you get too close to it. It grows in North America and Japan and is a member of the ginseng family (Araliaceae), as its genus name *Oplopanax* suggests. Though little used today and consequently difficult to obtain, it is an adaptogen that I have used with good results. It is mentioned here as 'one to watch' in the future, along with rose root. Incidentally, do not confuse devil's club with devil's claw; the latter is *Harpagophytum procumbens*, a Southern African herb used for arthritis.

Devil's club was used by several Native American tribes for a number of disorders, including arthritis, cancers, cataracts, coughs and colds, bronchitis and bleeding from the lungs, pain relief (stomach cramps and headaches) and rheumatism, as well as a general tonic. Herbalists in Canada use it as an adaptogen and it is certainly a herb worthy of further investigation. The bark, or root bark, is used, and the taste is reminiscent of *Panax ginseng*'s distinctive smoky bitter-sweetness.

**KEY ADAPTOGEN HERB**

# SIBERIAN GINSENG

**Scientific name** *Eleutherococcus senticosus*

**Plant family** Araliaceae (Ivy family)

**Type of plant** Tall deciduous shrub.

**Part used** Roots.

**Phytochemicals** Eleutherosides; triterpenoid saponins; glycans called eleutherans.

**Actions** Adaptogen, immune enhancer, tonic.

**Indications** Physical and mental stress, weakness and fatigue, to improve immune resistance.

**Preparations** Decoctions of the roots at a dosage of 1–2g per day for healthy adults; tincture prepared at a strength of 1:2 (where 1ml of tincture = 0.5g of dried Siberian ginseng roots) 2–4ml per day for healthy adults. (Higher doses may be used in treating disease states.) Take Siberian ginseng for six-week periods divided by two-week breaks.

**Combinations** As a general health aid it is best taken by itself.

**Cautions** Discontinue use during acute infections; recommence taking during the following recovery period.

**Conservation** Siberian ginseng is not considered to be a threatened species.

# PART III

# Weeks 4–6

At the end of Week 3, you will have reached a point where the foundations for your health transformation have been laid and these can now be built on. Part III looks at each system of the body and describes how to prevent disease and improve health in each of the systems, detailing which herbs to use to achieve these goals.

## Week 4

In Week 4, you will select your personal herbal allies to help improve your health in the areas where it needs it. Read Chapters 8–14, making notes as you do so, choosing up to three herbs to address your health needs. These three herbs should then be added to the antioxidant and adaptogen herbs you are taking which you chose in Weeks 2 and 3.

## Week 5

As well as describing the best herbs for each body system, Chapters 8–14 also describe the dietary, lifestyle and other measures that can improve your health. You should reflect on this advice and, where it seems important for your individual health, introduce it into your everyday life. During this week, you should continue to take your herbal mixture of antioxidant, adaptogen and herbal allies.

## Week 6 and beyond

Continue to take your herbal mixture until the end of Week 6. After this:

- Use the detoxification herbs periodically as required;
- Ensure there are sufficient antioxidants in your diet;
- Take herbal adaptogens periodically as required or take them in a continuing cycle (6 weeks taking the adaptogen followed by 2 weeks off) to enhance general functioning and prevent disease;
- Continue taking your herbal allies for as long as they are needed; return to this book for advice whenever you need extra help with your health;
- Maintain the positive dietary and lifestyle changes that you have found beneficial.

The 6 Week Herbal Detox Plan will always be there for you to consult in order to reflect on your health in the future and to offer you guidance on the best herbs to take and the best advice to follow.

# Chapter 8

# HERBS FOR THE IMMUNE SYSTEM –

## Enhancing resistance to illness

Developing and maintaining a healthy immune system is essential to achieving optimum health. Herbs that improve immune function have a huge role to play in assisting us to resist the threat of infections, and herbal medicine is supreme in priming the immune system to become swift and efficient in dealing with infection. Improved immune function can also help block the development of autoimmune diseases (diseases where the body attacks itself, such as rheumatoid arthritis and psoriasis), and it may contribute to the prevention of the development of some cancers.

The use of herbs in preventing or treating infectious disease is likely to become one of the main areas of interest for herbal practitioners in the coming years. One reason for this is that conventional medicine has severe limitations in this area and there are very few conventional drugs that successfully treat viral infections – the cause of illnesses such as the common cold. Secondly, it is becoming inappropriate to use conventional antibiotics to treat many of the infections that we develop because past excessive and inappropriate use of antibiotics has lead to the development of antibiotic-resistant micro-organisms ('super bugs'). There are now a number of organisms, such as methycillin-resistant *Staphylococcus aureus* (MRSA), that have become multi-antibiotic resistant and extremely hard to treat with conventional pharmaceuticals. Consequently, the use of antibiotics is increasingly limited to severe or life-threatening infections where they are crucial. Thankfully, most of the infections we encounter are of a less dramatic nature.

Medicinal plants are of particular value in preventing and treating infections because, in contrast to antibiotics, chemically they are very complex, making it difficult for infective organisms to adapt and become resistant to their influence.

Immune boosting herbs have another distinctive property in contrast with conventional drugs. Unlike the latter, herbs work alongside the normal actions of the immune system and help them to be more effective. In general, an infection will eventually burn itself out as the immune system gets to grips with it and brings it under control. The value of herbal immune agents is that they can speed up the rate at which the immune system deals with infections, so that we tend to get milder, less frequent and shorter-lived infections. By combining herbal immune enhancers with other improvements in our lifestyles, we may contract fewer infections and also be less prone to disease in general and cancer in particular. Appropriate lifestyle improvements include following a good wholefood diet with lots of fresh fruit and vegetables, reducing our stress levels, and achieving a balance between activity and rest – particularly regular exercise and good-quality sleep.

## The Immune System

Our bodies are well provided with mechanisms to help protect us from developing disease, especially infectious disease. The immune system is conventionally classified as having two major components:

- Innate immunity;
- Acquired immunity.

Acquired immunity can be further subdivided into two aspects:

- Humoral immunity;
- Cell-mediated immunity.

## Innate immunity

Innate immunity refers to the processes that provide the first line of immune defence. This includes basic mechanisms such as the barrier that the skin provides to prevent invasion of infection, and the antimicrobial activity of normal bodily secretions, such as tears, mucus and digestive enzymes. Innate immunity also includes a type of white blood cell called phagocytes, which are ready to respond to adverse micro-organisms. They attack infective organisms by wrapping around them and ingesting them. Other aspects of innate immunity include the 'complement complex' response by which a 'cascade' of proteins attacks invasive bacteria, and 'natural killer cells' (or 'natural killer lymphocytes') which can destroy infective micro-organisms and cancer cells. Innate immunity is sometimes called 'non-specific immunity' because it has general defensive properties across a broad spectrum of micro-organisms.

## Acquired immunity
### Humoral and cell-mediated immunity

Acquired immunity is developed over a period of time following exposure to infections. It is acquired by the creation of a specific response to particular types of micro-organism which manage to evade the innate immune system. The acquired system develops immune cells ('memory cells') that quickly recognise an infective agent that the body has been exposed to before and sends signals to other immune cells ('antibodies' and 'activated lymphocytes'), which rapidly multiply and attack the identified invader.

'Humoral immunity' is the development of antibodies and memory cells; it is known as B-cell immunity. 'Cell-mediated immunity' is the development of activated lymphocytes and memory cells; it is known as T-cell immunity.

So, when we encounter the chickenpox virus for the first time, it is too strong for our innate immunity to cope with and our acquired immunity is unable to recognise it so the infection establishes itself, leading to tiredness and the development of an itchy rash. As the

113

infection naturally dies out, the acquired immune system creates memory cells that can identify the virus the next time it is encountered and special antibodies that can disarm it before it has the chance to cause harm. As we live, grow and encounter each type of infective organism for the first time, our acquired immune system builds up a defence against the normal repertoire of infective diseases we may come across. This is why we would normally contract infections such as chickenpox and measles only once.

## Passive immunity

Lastly, there is 'passive immunity' that can be passed on to us from another individual who has developed acquired immunity to an organism that we have not yet encountered. The most typical way that passive immunity is achieved is through breastfeeding. Breast milk is a complex substance providing all the nutrients that a growing infant requires. It also contains immune enhancing substances, particularly antibodies, that the mother has developed, and the infant can make temporary use of these to protect them from disease. The newborn infant's immune system is weak and needs time to mature; breastfeeding provides cover for the baby's immune system until it is strong enough to deal with infections by itself and develop its own acquired immunity.

It is natural and healthy for children to develop infections after the initial period of high risk after birth and the acquired immunity built up in this way will mature the immune system, protecting us in later life. Infectious disease in children need not cause major health problems for children as long as they are well nourished and physically active before becoming ill and nursed carefully throughout the illness. It is appropriate that we develop infectious disease when we are young and have our parents or guardians around to care for us. When we are older, we cannot afford to be unwell because we have children of our own to care for and work to be done.

In children, herbal medicines work with the immune system to improve its response so that the initial degree of infection is mild to moderate rather than severe, and to help the rapid and effective development of acquired immunity to prevent further outbreaks of the disease. In adults, herbs can help to keep our immune defences strong, prevent them becoming weakened and depleted, and ensure that we continue to mount an effective challenge to disease organisms.

# Looking After Your Immune System

You may wonder why our immune system needs any help from herbal medicine, since it is clearly so well designed to protect us. The immune system will indeed perform effectively if nurtured with due care, but our natural immune functions can be weakened and their activities impaired by a number of internal and external influences. It is our goal to minimise these influences but this is not always easy once they have developed. In these circumstances, when the immune system is being undermined, herbal medicines have a vital part to play in helping our immune system to cope and to thrive. Below are some of the things that can reduce our immune system's capabilities.

## Poor diet

This can lead to the development of dietary deficiencies that leave us at increased risk of disease. White blood cells, the functional units of the immune system, can be weakened by deficiencies of vitamins A, C, E, B6 and B12, and by lack of folic acid and the minerals iron, zinc, manganese, copper and selenium. These same nutrients can boost immune function, especially vitamins C, E and B6, and selenium and zinc. A diet that impairs the immune system is one that is high in refined carbohydrates (white bread, cakes and biscuits), saturated fat and alcohol. Foods that enhance immune activity include fresh fruit and vegetables, whole grains, protein (such as fish and tofu), nuts and seeds, and essential fatty acids (such as those from sunflower oil and hemp oil).

## Lack of sleep

During sleep, the body repairs damaged cells and removes the accumulation of toxic products. The immune system is active in this process. Growth hormone is secreted during sleep to promote our physical development and sleep is considered to be very important in subconsciously dealing with psychological issues through dreaming. Chronic lack of sleep depletes our vital energy and diminishes the effectiveness of the immune system, leaving us at increased risk of becoming ill.

## Stress

Stress can be physical, emotional or mental both in origin and impact. In the West we live in a high-stress society where free time can be scarce and the demands of work and family life pronounced. The effects of stress may be exacerbated when we lack the traditional support network provided by a nearby extended family.

Prolonged stress can weaken immune performance, but pressure can be reduced by balancing active behaviour with a corresponding amount of restful or relaxing activities, developing good time-management strategies, removing unnecessary negative influences from our lives and developing a positive supportive group of personal contacts.

## Toxic exposure

Toxic chemicals can cause immune-system distress and overcome immune defences, causing damage to the body's tissues and organs. Severe toxic exposure often accompanies occupations such as coal mining and those involving working with asbestos. Both these substances can overwhelm the immune defences and lead to the development of cancer. There are also risks associated with occupations where there is regular work with lower grade toxic substances such as paints and solvents. Beyond this, we are all at some risk from toxic exposure at work and home from products such as cleaning and cosmetic preparations and 'air fresheners'. It is important to lower the burden on the immune system by avoiding toxic products in our homes.

## Immunosuppression

The immune system can be compromised by some illnesses and drugs. AIDS is perhaps the best-known disease that causes severe impairment of the immune system. People with AIDS can be exposed to such an extent, due to depletion of their immune resistance, that they can catch overwhelming infection from micro-organisms that would normally be relatively harmless. Some therapeutic drugs cause immune suppression but their use is necessary in certain circumstances, such as in preventing the rejection of organs in transplant patients. Lastly, it should be remembered that some recreational drugs, such as cocaine, can also lower immunity.

## Psychoneuroimmunology (PNI)

Immunity is also affected by our emotional responses, mental state and attitudes. The emerging discipline of psychoneuroimmunology (PNI, sometimes extended to psychoneuroendocrinoimmunology – PNEI), has shown us that links exist between our mind (psycho), our nervous system (neuro) and our immune state (immunology). It is also suggested that there are intimate links between these aspects and our hormonal system (endocrinology). It is clear that our immune resistance can be affected by what we feel and what we think. Those people who are clinically depressed have reduced immune activity, and people who are happy and content have increased immune activity. To achieve optimum immune function it is important to maintain a positive attitude of mind, while at the same time accepting our limitations and seeking help and support when we need it, rather than avoiding or burying difficult issues.

PNI is to do with our emotional and intellectual immunity, and our levels of immune resistance can be enhanced by a range of day-to-day activities that stimulate emotional and mental activity. This could include reading books, journals and newspapers; going to the cinema, theatre or gym; engaging in debate; playing games such as chess, bridge or crosswords; participating in social interactions and discussions; and involvement with art and nature.

## General advice

In addition to the above, the following advice will also help to promote immune health:

- Drink water regularly to moisten the mucous membranes and flush micro-organisms into the stomach where they can be destroyed by stomach acid.

- Get out into fresh air regularly. This is a tonic to the lungs and will help revitalise the immune system.

- Support liver function with the herbs referred to in Chapter 5 (*see* pages 71–2). The liver removes toxic products from the system, thereby reducing the demand on the immune system. The liver has its own specialised immune cells (Kuppfer cells) which are activated by liver stimulating herbs.

- Many of the adaptogen herbs mentioned in Chapter 7 have immune enhancing properties and can be taken in conjunction with the herbs described. The main difference between the adaptogenic herbs and the immune boosting herbs is that the adaptogens should not be taken during acute infections whereas the immune boosting herbs are ideally suited to this situation, as well as having disease-prevention properties.

- Add specific immune stimulating herbs/foods to your regular diet. Such plants could include lovage, beetroot, carrots, sweet potato, onion, garlic, thyme, watercress and nasturtium.

## Using immune-enhancing herbs

We all go through periods of time when our immune system needs support to help prevent us catching an infection or developing a disease. These are the stressful times when we have to work beyond the comfort zone of our normal capabilities and when we are unable to respond to our body's call to slow down or sleep. This can happen when we have deadlines to meet, or an unavoidable extra responsibility such as having to care for a sick relative. Positive events such as moving home or preparing for a wedding can also be stressful and cause our immune system to be stretched beyond its normal limits. Taking immune-enhancing herbs during these times can be very useful.

- We need to take extra immune herbs when we are exposed to extra risk – for example, when surrounded by colleagues, friends or relatives with colds; when working under extra pressure or in a polluted environment.

- People who work or play regularly with sources of low-level radiation such as computers and televisions are advised to improve their immune capacity with herbs, as are those working with toxic substances such as paints and solvents.

- If you tend to catch a lot of coughs and colds, continually being laid low by minor infections, you need to consider the issues discussed above and take herbal immune enhancers regularly.

- If you suffer from allergic conditions such as hay fever, asthma and eczema, your symptoms may improve by taking herbs that address the immune basis of these disorders.

- People who get recurrent infections such as chronic sinusitis, cystitis and vaginal thrush should consider taking immune boosting herbs, as should people with autoimmune diseases such as rheumatoid arthritis and ulcerative colitis.

Self-treatment with herbs to improve immune responses in times of stress or increased exposure to infection is frequently appropriate. However, if you suffer from an autoimmune condition (such as rheumatoid arthritis) you are advised to consult an experienced herbal practitioner to achieve the best possible results.

# Herbs for the Immune System

## Boneset

Boneset (*Eupatorium perfoliatum*) is a North American herb used
by Native American tribes for colds, flu, fevers, and as a general
tonic. It also relieves catarrhal congestion and is a mild laxative
– this herb might be particularly suitable if you tend to suffer
from constipation. It was used to repair broken bones by at least
one Native American tribe (the Abnaki), but its common name
probably derives from its use in treating so-called 'break-bone
fever' (now known as dengue, a mosquito-borne viral infection
which can cause severe joint and muscle pain). Alternatively,
the name may have to do with the fact that boneset was widely
used as a remedy for arthritis and rheumatism. It should not be
confused with knitbone (*Symphytum officinale*).

Boneset is a good herb to take when you are starting to feel
'under the weather' to help prevent the development of a fever,
or to treat one if it does it occur. The dried leaves should be used
as a tea made by infusion. Use 2 teaspoons per cup and drink 1
cup, 3–6 times a day from the first sign of an infection starting.

The European herb yarrow (*Achillea millefolium*) has similar
attributes and indications to boneset and can be used in the
same way. However, it should not be taken in pregnancy.

## Cat's claw

Cat's claw (*Uncaria tomentosa*) is a South and Central American
vine with small, claw-like thorns that has been used by Peruvian
tribes for at least 2,000 years. As well as being an immune-
system stimulant, it has long been used to treat asthma, arthritis,
rheumatism and cancer. This plant may be of particular use if
you suffer from any of these conditions. It contains alkaloids
which boost the levels of the immune-system constituents called

interleukins. Interleukins act as mediators of the immune response, causing an increase in the number of immune cells such as the large white blood cells known as macrophages that can engulf and destroy up to 100 bacteria at a time, as well as organisms as large as the parasites that cause malaria.

The vine or root bark is used and should be taken as a tea made by decoction. Use 2 teaspoons to a cup and take 1 cup each day.

## Chiretta (andrograpis)

This plant, like echinacea, is better known by its botanical name (*Andrographis paniculata*) than its common name. Andrographis is a shrub occurring in India and is used in Ayurvedic and traditional Chinese medicine. It is a very useful immune stimulant that particularly increases the number of phagocytes – small white blood cells that attack invading micro-organisms. It tastes quite bitter and, like most bitter herbs, tends to improve liver function and the digestion. If you have a poor appetite and digestion or are prone to develop skin infections, this herb may suit you particularly well. It is very good to use if you experience recurrent colds or sore throats.

Due to its bitterness, this herb is better taken as a tincture or tablet rather than as a tea – unless you happen to like bitter tasting drinks! The tincture dosage for regular use of andrographis is 4–6 ml per day of the 1:2 strength preparation. This herb is considered to be very safe, but should be avoided in pregnancy.

## Echinacea (coneflower)

The common name of this plant is coneflower due to the presence of a pronounced dome or cone formation in the centre of the flower head. The naturally occurring *Echinacea* species come in varying shades of purple; the most commonly used species is *Echinacea purpurea* with strongly purple-pink petals, while *Echinacea pallida* is so called because of the pale purple-pink colour of its petals. Several ornamental varieties exist with different-coloured flowers, especially yellow and white, but only the true purple petal species are used in medicine. The botanical name *Echinacea* derives from the Greek word for hedgehog (*echinos*) which refers to the spiky, prickly nature of the central cone. The main active constituents in tea or tincture preparations are the alkylamides – it is these that cause the characteristic tingling sensation that echinacea stimulates on the tongue.

Much of the research into echinacea has been conducted on purified and stabilised polysaccharide fractions from the fresh flower head given to people by intravenous injection, so although this research has achieved a wide influence, it cannot be taken as representing the effects of traditional root preparations (which are very low in polysaccharides) given to people by mouth.

Echinacea is a most valuable immune stimulant and is probably the most widely used medicinal herb in complementary medicine in the West today. Its major impact on the immune system, like that of andrographis, is to stimulate the phagocyte cells and these are the first line of immune defence. Echinacea can be used to prevent and treat the common cold and other viral, bacterial and fungal infections. It typically reduces the frequency of colds and, if they do occur, it decreases their duration and severity. If you are prone to recurrent colds, coughs, chest infections, thrush, allergies or skin diseases such as acne and boils, echinacea may be of great benefit to you.

It can be taken long term to improve the condition of your immune system if you live or work in an unhealthy or polluted environment. If you suffer from hay fever, start taking echinacea a month before the time of year when your symptoms usually start. If you tend to have recurrent winter colds, start taking echinacea just before winter begins and keep taking it throughout the season.

Echinacea can be taken in various forms but the best is probably as a tea or a tincture. Prepare the tea by decoction, using 3 teaspoons to a cup, and take 1 cup a day for general preventive purposes and 3–4 cups if an acute infection occurs. Take 3–9ml per day of the 1:2 tincture for general preventive purposes and double this amount for an acute infection.

## Elderflower and elderberries

The elder (*Sambucus nigra*) is a small tree that has been used in medicine in Europe for many centuries. The flowers are creamy white and have a pleasant taste and odour when dried and used as a tea. They stimulate the immune response and have anticatarrhal and anti-allergic properties. They make an excellent drink to take regularly through the autumn and winter seasons to ward off colds, and can be spiced up by adding a few cloves and a little cinnamon. Elderflower tea can be very helpful if you suffer from hay fever or mucus congestion problems. It also helps to reduce joint and muscle pains, so providing appropriate immune enhancement if you experience these problems.

Elderberries are small, purple-black fruits that appear in clusters on the tree. A study has shown that they improve the rate of recovery from influenza infection. The berries enhance immune activity and contain antioxidants that may help to prevent cancer. They are particularly helpful as an immune stimulant during periods of fatigue or when convalescing after an illness because their nutrient content (including vitamins A and C) helps the body to be restored to health.

The flowers are best taken as a tea; use 2 teaspoons of the dried
flowers per cup and prepare by infusion. Take 1–2 cups a day for
general immune enhancing effects and 3–4 cups a day in acute infections. Commercial preparations of the juice concentrate are available or, if you have access to elder trees, you can collect the berries
and make them into a fruit preserve for use as part of your diet.

## Marigold

Marigold (*Calendula officianalis*) is a beautiful orange flower that
is easy and rewarding to grow. It contains glycosides and resins,
both of which have immune stimulating properties. In addition,
it has excellent anti-inflammatory and wound-healing properties.
Marigold is particularly useful to take for optimising immune
functions if you suffer from skin infections (such as acne, boils
and ringworm) or inflammatory bowel disease. It may also be a
good herb to use if you tend to have congested menstrual periods
with pain. It can also be helpful if you are subject to food
intolerance or allergies; the healing effect of marigold on the wall
of the digestive system combined with its anti-inflammatory and
immunostimulant actions can be of great assistance here.

Marigold is best taken as a tea made by infusion. Use 1 teaspoon
of the petals to a cup and take 2–3 cups a day to improve immune
function. Teas extract the water-soluble glycosides from the
flowers but do not extract the resins. The resins stimulate
leucocytosis (an increase in white blood cells) and have effects on
bacterial and fungal infections. A tincture made with 90% alcohol
and 10% water will extract the resins effectively, but this type of
concentrated preparation is more appropriate for professional use.

## Pau d'arco

Pau d'arco (*Tabebuia* species) is a majestic South American tree
with striking tubular flowers. The bark is the part used

medicinally and this is harvested from several different species of the tree, with the pink to purple flowered species being preferred to those with yellow flowers. It has antiviral, antifungal and anticancer properties, and has been used as part of the treatment for serious immune disorders such as cancer, leukaemia and HIV/AIDS. You may find it helpful if you suffer from *Candida* infection (thrush), eczema, psoriasis, cold sores, genital herpes or chronic fatigue syndrome.

Although pau d'arco is used in the treatment of very severe disorders, it is also suitable for boosting general immunity. For this purpose, take either the bark made into a tea by decoction, or the tincture. For the tea, use 2 teaspoons of the bark and drink 1 cup a day. With the tincture, the 1:2 strength is taken at a dose of 3–7ml per day.

## St John's wort

St John's wort (*Hypericum perforatum*) is dealt with in more detail in Chapter 14 where its effects on the mood are discussed (*see* pages 246–7). It is included here because it has an immune-system function as an antiviral agent. It is particularly effective against enveloped viruses, including those that cause cold sores, shingles, chickenpox, genital herpes, glandular fever and viral hepatitis. Considering the link between mind, emotions and immune health, St John's wort may be particularly helpful if you suffer from a combination of depressed mood and low immune function.

This herb can interact with several important drugs and you should consult a herbal practitioner and your doctor before taking it if you are using a strong conventional drug on which your health depends.

Take St John's wort as a tea made by infusion at a dose of 2 teaspoons to a cup with 1 cup drunk 2–3 times a day.

## KEY HERB FOR THE IMMUNE SYSTEM

# ECHINACEA

**Scientific name** *Echinacea* species. Several different species are used medicinally. *E. purpurea* is used most commonly, followed by *E. angustifolia* and *E. pallida*.

**Plant family** Asteraceae (Daisy family)

**Type of plant** Perennial herb.

**Part used** Mainly the roots, sometimes the flowering tops and occasionally the whole plant.

**Phytochemicals** Alkylamides; caffeic acid esters (echinacoside, chicoric acid); volatile oil.

**Actions** Immunostimulant; anti-inflammatory; lymphatic; vulnerary.

**Indications** Immunodeficiency states; as an adjunctive treatment in cancer therapy; coughs, colds, flu; allergic and autoimmune diseases; suppurative skin diseases – acne, abscesses, boils.

**Preparations** Tincture (1:2) – take 3–9ml per day for general preventative purposes but increase this dose by 2–3 times for a short period (3–7 days) if an acute infection arises. You can also prepare a tea from the roots by decoction – take 1.5–4.5g per day for preventative purposes and increase this by a factor of 2–3 times in acute infections.

**Combinations** Can be taken by itself.

**Cautions** Echinacea is generally well tolerated and safe. If you have an immunosuppressive disease or are taking immunosuppressive drugs (such as those used by organ transplant patients) you should seek expert advice before taking this herb.

**Conservation** *E. purpurea* is widely cultivated for medicinal use and its use presents no ecological concerns. It is important to use only cultivated and not wild-harvested *E. angustifolia* plants. Some species of *Echinacea* are endangered (such as *E. tennesseensis*) but they are not used in medicine.

# Chapter 9

# HERBS FOR THE DIGESTIVE SYSTEM –

## The platform of health

The digestive system is essentially a long, convoluted tube stretching from the mouth to the anus. This tube, also known as the alimentary tract, is about 9 metres (30ft) long in an adult; much of this length is coiled in the small intestines. The alimentary tract is supplied with various secretions that assist in the breakdown and absorption of food from the accessory organs of digestion, including the salivary glands, liver, gall bladder and pancreas. Overall control of the digestive system is via the nervous system and hormonal control centres. The primary functions of the digestive system are to absorb water and vital nutrients and to excrete waste products. The digestive process keeps the body nourished, providing the materials and energy for the body to grow and perform.

Herbal medicines can have powerful actions in promoting digestive health and optimal functioning. There is an important interaction with herbs when working with the digestive system because most herbs are taken by mouth and come into direct contact with the surface of the alimentary tract as they are processed. This provides an opportunity for herbs to have profound and rapid effects in treating diseases of the intestines as well as improving the natural work of this area of the body. Herbs can improve food processing, digestion and absorption in the digestive system, reduce inflammation, soothe and relax, and promote healing of damaged tissue.

The digestive system provides the foundation for health since the body cannot achieve perfect health without an effective digestive system to supply it with the fuel it needs to thrive and to remove the waste products that would otherwise cause congestion and disruption of normal functions.

# The Digestive System

## Mouth

The mouth is involved in breaking up and chewing food so that it is ready to be swallowed. Mouth ulcers can have a number of causes, including digestive system diseases (such as ulcerative colitis and coeliac disease) and nutritional deficiencies (iron, folic acid and vitamin B12), though in many cases no specific causes can be found, in which case it is likely that the ulcers are a sign of depleted immunity. Nutritional deficiency is also suggested by cracking in the corners of the mouth (angular stomatitis). Dental problems, including poorly fitting dentures, can impair chewing and therefore digestive function. Gum inflammation (gingivitis) is usually due to bacterial infection.

## Salivary glands

The salivary glands keep the mouth moist and secrete enzymes which begin the process of breaking down food once it enters the mouth. The mouth can become dry due to suppression of salivary gland activity in anxiety states and during a fever. Some drugs and certain diseases can also cause this problem. Infection of the parotid salivary glands is known as mumps.

## Oesophagus

The oesophagus lies behind the trachea (windpipe) and is a more or less straight tube that provides a channel for food and fluids to pass from the mouth to the stomach. It secretes mucus to ease the passage of food and has a sphincter at its lower end which releases food into the stomach. Disorders of the oesophagus may cause difficulty in swallowing. The most common oesophageal problem is heartburn (reflux oesophagitis), which results from movement of stomach acid into the oesophagus. This problem can be very painful and is made worse by lying flat or bending over as this tilts the acid into the oesophagus. The pain can spread from the oesophagus to the chest, neck and arms, and can be mistaken for the pain of heart disease.

## Stomach

The stomach breaks down food by grinding it mechanically by muscular contractions and chemically by secreting hydrochloric acid and enzymes such as pepsin. The stomach is extremely acidic (pH 2) and the stomach walls are specially constructed to resist the potentially destructive effects of its own secretions. (To get an idea of how acidic stomach acid is, if you spilt it on your hand it would burn through it!) The stomach does not absorb nutrients, but some water, a few drugs and alcohol can be absorbed into the bloodstream through it. Commonly encountered stomach problems include inflammation (gastritis) and ulcers (particularly due to infection with *Helicobacter pylori*).

## Pancreas

The pancreas secretes pancreatic juice containing water, salts, sodium bicarbonate and enzymes into the duodenum (the short tube that connects the stomach with the small intestine). Pancreatic juice is alkaline and it neutralises stomach acid as it passes down into the small intestine. The pancreatic enzymes help break down the proteins, carbohydrates and fats in food. The pancreas also secretes hormones that operate outside the digestive system; chief amongst these is insulin, which is vital in the metabolism of sugars in the blood. The pancreas can be affected by inflammatory disease (pancreatitis) and this may be either acute or chronic in nature.

## Liver and gall bladder

The liver is an organ which performs many different functions including:

- Metabolism of carbohydrates, fats and proteins;
- Detoxification of drugs and hormones;
- Storage of vitamins, minerals and sugars;
- Activation of vitamin D;
- Immune functions.

The liver's most significant contribution to the digestive system is in synthesising bile salts and then excreting this as bile into the gall bladder. The gall bladder then releases bile into the small intestine when food is passing into it. Bile salts enable the emulsification and absorption of fats, including cholesterol.

The liver can be affected by many diseases, including hepatitis and cirrhosis. The gall bladder can be affected by gall stones (most commonly made from cholesterol) and inflammation (cholecystitis).

## Small intestine

The small intestine is narrower than the large intestine but much longer. It stretches from the stomach to the large intestine and is coiled to fit into the abdomen. It secretes a slightly alkaline juice that aids the further breakdown of food constituents to a point where they are ready to be absorbed. The majority of nutrient and water absorption occurs in the small intestine, particularly in the final third of its length. Disorders of the small intestine include malabsorption syndromes, coeliac disease (sensitivity to gluten from wheat and some other grains) and Crohn's disease. Food intolerance and allergies may result from the abnormal absorption of food products across the small intestine, leading to an autoimmune response occurring every time the food is eaten; this is known as 'leaky gut syndrome'.

## Large intestine

The large intestine, or large bowel, carries out further absorption of
food and water and it removes waste products from the body via the
faeces. The last stage of digestion in the large intestine is enabled
by bacteria rather than enzymes and so it is essential to maintain a
healthy bowel flora of beneficial bacteria. Conditions affecting the
large intestine include:

- Constipation,
- Diarrhoea,
- Haemorrhoids,
- Ulcerative colitis,
- Diverticulitis,
- Irritable bowel syndrome,
- Cancer.

# Caring for your digestive system

There are a number of things that you can do to improve your
digestive health in addition to taking herbs. The most useful ones
are set out below.

**Eat and drink regularly** – The digestive system works best with a
regular eating pattern. Always eat breakfast and remember that
eating little and often is better than eating large meals infrequently.

**Make time to eat** – We need to be relaxed and restful in order for the
body to devote its efforts towards digestion and not have to help us
perform other physical activities. Try not to rush your food; it is
important that you chew food thoroughly – it will not be digested
properly if it has not been properly prepared in the mouth. Try to
make at least one meal a day a family or social event; avoid eating
in front of the TV and engage in conversation instead.

**Drink enough water** – It is important to drink water regularly and in adequate amounts. Water requirements vary depending on your body weight and the ambient temperature, but are normally 1.5–2 litres a day for the average adult. Make water your main drink of the day. Try not to go more than one hour without having a drink.

**Encourage regular motions** – We talk about 'bowel habits' and so they are. Bowel movements are not an instinctive but a learned behaviour. Try and get into good bowel habits not bad ones. Listen to 'the call of nature' and respond immediately; avoid holding on to motions and delaying going to the toilet because eventually the body will follow your lead and suppress the natural urge to defecate. This is one of the most common causes of chronic constipation. Conventional medical texts generally state that the normal frequency of bowel movements ranges from three times a day to once every three days. Herbalists believe that a bowel movement at least once every day is an important sign of general health.

**Avoid using strong laxatives and antacids** – Many pharmacy drugs of this type can cause damage to the digestive system and promote dependency. If you suffer from chronic constipation or acidity, visit a herbal practitioner for corrective treatment and use foods such as figs, plums and prunes to help ease the motions instead of drugs.

**Ensure there is a regular supply of soluble fibre in the diet** –Many people supplement their diets with harsh insoluble fibre, especially in the form of wheat bran, and this often causes irritation to the gastrointestinal tract. Instead of this, use soluble fibre, such as that provided abundantly in the skins of fruits (as pectins) and in some grains such as oat bran. Soluble fibre is gentle and well tolerated, and helps to promote regular comfortable bowel movements. By improving the frequency of bowel movements, the time that carcinogens contained in the diet have to make contact with the bowel wall is reduced, and so is the risk of developing bowel cancer. Bowel cancer is one of the most common forms of cancer in the West, although it is not as well known as some other forms, possibly because many people are sensitive about discussing bowel movements. Soluble fibre also helps to mop up excess cholesterol in the diet and so has an important role to play in preventing high cholesterol and the heart disease that is associated with it. Good sources of soluble fibre include fruits (especially the skins of fruits such as apples, peaches, pears), vegetables (including broccoli, spinach and vegetables with their skins such as carrots, parsnips and potatoes), legumes such as kidney beans and lentils, and cereals such as oat bran.

**Eat a wholefood diet and avoid congestive and irritating foods** – A wholefood diet means one that is high in fresh fruit, vegetables and whole grains, and low in refined and processed foods such as white flour, sugar, and ready-cooked meals. Such a diet is naturally rich in soluble fibre and will improve bowel tone and promote regular motions. It will also be rich in cancer-preventive antioxidants.

**Avoid excessive exposure to tannins** – Tannins are plant chemicals that come in several forms. Some are valuable antioxidants while others can bind to iron in foods and prevent it from being adequately absorbed. Such binding tannins are present in black Chinese or Indian tea, so it is a good idea to avoid an excessive intake of this beverage. Green tea has more potent antioxidant activity than black tea but alternatives that are low in iron-binding tannins are preferable. Such teas, which can be regularly consumed in place of 'ordinary' tea, include the leaves of the South African shrubs rooibos (also known as red bush) and mountain honeybush.

**Avoid toxins taken by mouth** – This includes artificial food additives that may cause injury to the digestive system or act as carcinogens, and drugs such as aspirin and other nonsteroidal anti-inflammatory drugs (NSAIDs), which can cause bleeding from the stomach, and paracetamol, which can cause liver damage. Use herbal medicines as alternatives.

**Optimise the natural bowel flora** – This can be done by regular consumption of soluble fibre and live natural yoghurt, and by avoiding antibiotics unless essential. Probiotic products are available which contain live bacteria; these can be used to help repopulate the bowel with 'friendly' micro-organisms after antibiotic use or at other times when such support is needed.

**Carry out regular detoxification** – This can help cleanse the system and clear out waste products, revitalising the digestive system. (*See* Chapter 5 for more on detoxification.)

**Take regular physical exercise** – A sedentary lifestyle carries a higher risk of chronic constipation. Regular physical exercise helps to improve circulation to the digestive system and enhance its tone and performance. It also reduces the likelihood of developing haemorrhoids. In particular, pelvic floor exercises will help to prevent haemorrhoids: clench your buttocks together as if trying to hold in wind for 2 seconds then relax again; repeat this 10 times in a row and do it several times a day.

**Be careful with early feeding of children** – The small intestines of infants are more porous than those of adults and can absorb large proteins that may set up an immune response leading to an allergic response to foods containing them in later life. This particularly applies to the large proteins present in wheat and dairy products. It is important to avoid giving wheat- or dairy-based foods to children until after they are 12 months old. By this time, the digestive system will have developed sufficiently to cope with such foods if they are introduced gradually and in moderate amounts.

## Herbal Actions on the Digestive System

Before looking in detail at the most useful individual herbs for the digestive system it is useful to look at the actions that herbs can have.

## Antacid

Several herbs can act to reduce excess acidity. Such herbs can be useful if you experience digestive problems such as heartburn or gastritis. Angelica (*Angelica archangelica*) and sweet flag (*Acorus calamus*) are among the most useful herbs here, and marshmallow root (*Althea officinalis*) and slippery elm (*Ulmus rubra*) are also of value since they coat the gut with a soothing mucilage.

## Antiemetic

Antiemetics are herbs that reduce nausea; these include ginger (*Zingiber officinalis*) and peppermint (*Mentha piperita*).

## Anti-inflammatory

Herbs reducing inflammation in the gastrointestinal tract include marigold (*Calendula officinalis*), liquorice (*Glycyrrhiza glabra*) and meadowsweet (*Filipendula ulmaria*). They are used in the treatment of diverticulitis and inflammatory bowel disorders such as ulcerative colitis. They are also important in relieving indigestion.

## Antispasmodic

Antispasmodic herbs promote the relaxation of the muscles of the alimentary tract and help to ease pain and discomfort. Herbs that have this activity can help reduce flatulence and constipation; such herbs include chamomile (*Matricaria recutita*) and ginger (*Zingiber officinalis*).

## Astringent

Astringents bind tissues and secretions and are particularly helpful for those prone to loose bowel movements or diarrhoea. They can also be effective in treating mouth ulcers when used as a mouthwash. Gentle but reliable digestive astringents include agrimony (*Agrimonia eupatorium*) and blackberry leaf (*Rubus fruticosus*).

## Bitters

Bitter herbs (bitters) stimulate saliva production, stomach acid and digestive enzymes. They also cause the liver to produce bile. These actions can combine to help improve digestion by improving the breakdown and absorption of nutrients. Bitters also stimulate the appetite and have a mild laxative effect (bile is an aperient or gentle laxative in its own right). By improving stomach acid production, bitters can play an important role in resisting infection since we rely on optimum stomach acidity to destroy ingested infective agents, especially bacteria. Taking drops of bitters before meals can be useful when travelling to prevent infection, as well as maintaining healthy digestive and bowel functions. If you have difficulty with fatty foods, bitters enhance bile production, so improving the emulsification of fats. Excellent bitter herbs include wormwood (*Artemisia absinthium*) – but do not take it during pregnancy – quassia (*Picrasma excelsa*) and centaury (*Centaurium erythrea*).

Aromatic bitters are herbs that combine bitter properties with volatile oil content. As a consequence they are both stimulating (due to the bitters) and relaxing (due to the volatile oils). They also stimulate local circulation, producing a warming and soothing response. Aromatic bitters are excellent for improving cold or sluggish digestion, and for relieving chronic indigestion, griping pain and flatulence. One of the best in this category of herbs is cinnamon (*Cinnamomum zeylanicum*).

## Carminative

Carminative herbs are rich in volatile oils and they warm and relax the small and large intestines. They are calming and relaxing to the bowel, and are useful for flatulence and spasmodic digestive pain. Important carminatives include aniseed (*Pimpinella anisum*), angelica (*Angelica archangelica*), caraway (*Carum carvi*) and fennel (*Foeniculum vulgare*).

## Demulcent

Demulcent herbs have the ability to form gel-like preparations when mixed with water and these will coat the lining of the alimentary tract. This creates a soothing barrier over inflamed tissues and areas of increased acidity. Demulcents are tremendously helpful in inflammatory conditions of the digestive system such as heartburn.

## Laxative

Laxatives promote bowel movements and herbal laxatives can be placed in one of two groups: stimulating laxatives and bulk-forming laxatives. The former group have a stimulant effect on bile production or on muscular movements of the bowel and includes herbs such as burdock (*Arctium lappa*) and cascara sagrada (*Rhamnus purshiana*). Bulk-forming laxatives have a gentler action and work by swelling in the bowel and gently triggering bowel movements while also lubricating the motions. Examples of these include psyllium seeds (*Plantago psyllium*) and linseeds (*Linum usitatissimum*).

## Mental and emotional relaxants

Antispasmodics and carminatives both have relaxant effects on the muscles of the digestive system, but some herbs promote gastrointestinal relaxation from a higher level of the nervous system as they cause relaxation of the mind. There are strong connections between the digestive system and the mind and emotions – when we are anxious we may talk of having 'butterflies in the stomach', and anxiety can cause some people to keep rushing to the toilet before, say, an examination or stage performance. Some people have a digestion that is easily disrupted by their mental or emotional state; this is one of the factors involved in irritable bowel syndrome. If you are prone to a sensitive, easily disrupted bowel, then relaxants that influence the bowel from an emotional or mental level can be very useful; examples include valerian (*Valeriana officinalis*), hops (*Humulus lupulus*) and chamomile (*Matricaria recutita*).

# Herbs for the Digestive System

Regular use of these herbs will help to enhance the performance of the digestive system and protect it from damage and disease. Rotation of herbal teas such as peppermint, chamomile, fennel, dandelion and marshmallow, alongside dietary use of cinnamon and daily consumption of linseeds and slippery elm, will provide excellent digestive support.

## Caraway and fennel

Seeds from several medicinal plants in the Apiaceae (formerly the Umbelliferae) family have antispasmodic and carminative properties. Prime among these are caraway (*Carum carvi*), fennel (*Foeniculum vulgare*), angelica (*Angelica archangelica*) and aniseed (*Pimpinella anisum*). Seeds from caraway and another Apiaceae family member, dill (*Anethum graveolens*), are traditional ingredients in gripe water, which is used to relieve colic (spasm of the intestines) in children. Caraway and fennel are excellent to take as teas if you are prone to experiencing abdominal tightness, bloating or trapped wind. By improving circulation to the bowel they are warming and relaxing and promote bowel comfort and ease of motions. Take 1 cup of tea made by infusing 2 teaspoons of the seeds as required. You can also buy tea bags containing fennel but if you are using the raw seeds, it helps to release the volatile oils if you bruise them in a pestle and mortar first.

## Chamomile

Chamomile (*Matricaria recutita*) is sometimes referred to as 'the mother of the gut'. It reduces inflammation and spasm of the muscles in the digestive system, these actions combining to relieve pain and tenderness. The relaxant effect of chamomile complements a slight bitterness in taste that stimulates bile flow; together these activities help to promote healthy bowel movements. In spite of the mild bitterness, chamomile is a very pleasant and refreshing drink; the agreeable taste and gentle yet significant effects on the digestion make chamomile one of the most popular of all herbal teas. Chamomile is healing to the gut wall as it stimulates the formation of new tissue over areas of erosion in the lining of the alimentary tract; it also has a mild sedative activity (Peter Rabbit drank chamomile tea to help him sleep!), which reduces the impact that our emotions and mental state have on the bowel.

Chamomile is a truly marvellous herb that is widely available in teabag form (try and choose organic brands), but it can also be made from the loose flowers by using 2 teaspoons to a cup and infusing for 5–10 minutes. Drink this tea hot, savouring it and inhaling the lovely volatile oil as you do so. Drinking a cup before bed will help you sleep, particularly if you are sometimes kept awake by abdominal tenderness.

## Cinnamon

Cinnamon (*Cinnamomum zeylanicum*) is a well-known culinary spice used particularly in desserts and confectionery. Few people know that it is also an important medicinal herb. It is an aromatic bitter having both relaxing and stimulant effects on the digestion. It warms the digestive circulation and relaxes tension in the abdomen. It also has antimicrobial activity, particularly against infective bacteria including *Helicobacter pylori*, the bacteria that causes the majority of stomach ulcers. This property makes cinnamon valuable in the treatment of food poisoning. It is a good herb to use if you tend to suffer from loose motions, including as part of irritable bowel syndrome.

Take cinnamon as a decoction of the bark (often sold as 'quills') – use 2 teaspoons of crushed bark (break it up in a pestle and mortar) to a cup and take a cup as required.

# Dandelion

Dandelion root (*Taraxacum officinale*) is an excellent herb to support the digestive function. Its major impact is due to its tonic effect on the liver. Dandelion has a stimulating effect on liver cells (hepatocytes), improving their general functions and enhancing bile production, leading to a mild laxative influence. It also improves the absorption of nutrients from food and the detoxification of alcohol by the liver.

Take dandelion root as a decoction: use 2 teaspoons of the dried chopped roots to a cup and drink a cup as required. Roasted dandelion root is also available as 'dandelion coffee' and this can also be used but it requires one word of caution – some dandelion coffee brands have lactose added and you should avoid them if you are sensitive to milk products.

# Linseeds

Linseeds (*Linum usitatissimum*) are the most useful of the bulk-forming laxatives. To use them for this purpose, take 2 teaspoons to 1 dessertspoon of the raw whole (not dehulled) seeds each morning with water. Take the seeds sprinkled on your breakfast cereal or mixed in a cup of water or juice. Whichever method you use, it is very important that you wash the seeds down with two further full glasses of water. This is because the seeds need to swell up in the bowel in order to bulk up and ease bowel movements, and they can only do this if they have enough water to absorb as they sit in the bowel. I stress this point because many people take linseeds by soaking the seeds in water overnight and then drinking the resulting gel that forms in the morning. This method is excellent if you have heartburn because the demulcent gel will soothe the oesophagus, but it has no significant laxative effect. The seeds need to swell up *in* the bowel, not outside it. It is important to use seeds that have not been dehulled because the husks act as an 'enteric coating', helping the seeds pass in to the bowel intact and not be metabolised by stomach acid.

Linseeds are excellent for long-term daily use because they possess several other benefits in addition to improving bowel movements. By reducing the time that the bowel is exposed to carcinogens from the diet and the metabolism, they may help prevent bowel cancer. They are rich in soluble fibre and help to bind cholesterol, thus reducing the risk of heart disease. They also contain omega 3 essential fatty acids, often deficient in diets in the West. These help to promote a healthy fat profile in the body and they nourish the skin and prevent inflammatory disease. Additionally, they contain phytoestrogenic lignans, which are helpful in controlling the menopause, and they may have a role in preventing oestrogen-dependent tumours such as breast cancer in women and prostrate cancer in men.

## Marshmallow

Most of us think of marshmallows as sticky sweets, but there are medicinal origins to this product. The leaves, roots and flowers of the marshmallow plant (Althaea officinalis) contain sugar chains called polysaccharides which mix with water to form a soothing gel that is excellent in reducing stomach acidity, coating and protecting areas of inflammation in the digestive tract and relieving heartburn. A preparation was formerly made, part confection and part medicine, combining the roots of marshmallow with sugar to produce a sweet that was taken for sore throats and chests, coughs and hoarseness. The modern-day 'marshmallows' derive from this product but no longer contain marshmallow itself and are no longer therapeutic items.

Regularly drinking a decoction of marshmallow roots can be valuable if you suffer from heartburn, excessive stomach acidity or any kind of inflammatory digestive disease. They are generally soothing and calming for sore or tense digestive systems, and will gently help to promote normal tone and function in this area. Use 2 teaspoons to a cup and drink as required.

## Peppermint

Peppermint (*Mentha piperita*) is a well-known and widely-used herbal tea that is readily available in teabag form. It is a wonderful herb for the digestive system, having a number of beneficial effects. It relieves spasm and calms tension in the alimentary tract. It also increases bile production, thereby encouraging healthy bowel movements. This may be the herb for you if you tend to experience indigestion, irritable bowel syndrome, flatulence, mild constipation, digestive tightness and pain, bloating of the abdomen or nausea. Additionally, peppermint has effects outside the digestive system in treating headaches, fevers, colds and bronchitis.

Peppermint has a slightly stimulating effect on the nervous system, so it can provide an alternative to coffee if you are trying to cut down or give up but find you miss the energy kick that it gives. This quality also means that peppermint should not be drunk excessively (take no more than 2–3 cups a day, alternating with other teas such as chamomile). It is best avoided last thing at night in case it interferes with normal sleep.

Take peppermint as an infusion either of a teabag or of the loose chopped leaves at a dose of 1–2 teaspoons per cup.

## Slippery elm

Slippery elm is a pink powder scraped from the inner surface of the bark from a species of North American elm tree (*Ulmus rubra*). It is called slippery because if you mix the powder with water it swells up to form a slippery gel (also called 'slippery elm gruel') that has strong demulcent qualities. This preparation is excellent for soothing the digestive system in cases of inflammation and irritation. It is particularly used to offset the effects of heartburn. It can also help to soften the stools, making them easier and more comfortable to pass.

You should consider using slippery elm if you tend to heartburn, soreness in the abdomen or hard stools. It has also been used as a nourishing and nurturing food in periods of convalescence, and is worth trying if you are experiencing feelings of weakness, depletion and fatigue.

Take slippery elm as 1 dessertspoon of the raw powder mixed slowly with enough water to form a watery gel and then drunk. This can be taken as often as required and is best taken before meals if you have heartburn or acidity problems. Tablets are also available which can be taken with water. They will then swell up in the stomach and intestines, releasing their healing influence.

## KEY HERB FOR THE DIGESTIVE SYSTEM

## CHAMOMILE
(also known as **German chamomile**)

**Scientific name** *Matricaria recutita*

**Plant family** Asteraceae (Daisy family)

**Type of plant** Annual herb.

**Part used** Flowers.

**Phytochemicals** Flavonoids; volatile oil – containing bisabolol and chamazulene.

**Actions** Anti-inflammatory, antimicrobial, antispasmodic, gentle sedative, vulnerary.

**Indications** General relaxant and soothing for the digestive system. Used for spasmodic pain, diarrhoea, flatulence, nausea, travel sickness, inflammatory bowel disorders.

**Preparations** Best taken as a tea. Use 2 teaspoons to a cup and prepare as an infusion. Drink 1–4 cups a day as required.

**Combinations** Combines well with a number of herbs, including peppermint and meadowsweet.

**Cautions** Chamomile is very safe, gentle and well tolerated, but some people find the smell and taste slightly nauseating.

**Conservation** *Matricaria recutita* is widely cultivated for medicinal use and its use presents no ecological concerns.

# Chapter 10

# HERBS FOR THE CARDIOVASCULAR SYSTEM –

## How to maintain a healthy heart

The heart and the blood vessels (arteries and veins) go to make up the body's cardiovascular system. One of the main purposes of the cardiovascular system is to supply the organs and tissues of the body with oxygen, while removing carbon dioxide from the body, and this purpose is achieved through the circulation of the blood.

In ancient medicine and up to the nineteenth century, blood-letting was one of the major therapeutic medical procedures. Physicians believed that congestion of the blood led to many kinds of disease and that regular easing of stagnation by drawing off the blood promoted good health. It was not until the seventeenth century that William Harvey first demonstrated how blood flows around the body. He showed that the heart acted as a pump and that the blood was in constant motion around the body. Until then it had been widely believed that blood was contained within specific areas of the body and did not circulate all the way around. Blood is one of the four humours of ancient medicine (*see* page 8) and was described as being hot and moist in nature and associated with the element of air. It was believed that the blood contained air (*pneuma*). This showed a rudimentary appreciation of the oxygen-carrying capacity that is one of the major attributes of blood.

# The Circulatory System

When we breathe in, air is taken deep into the lungs, where oxygen is absorbed into the blood and carbon dioxide is released into the lungs to be discharged from the body during expiration. In this way the blood both absorbs oxygen and expels the waste product of oxygen metabolism, carbon dioxide. Oxygen, carried in the blood by combining with haemoglobin in the red blood cells, is essential in all the body's cells for the production of energy.

The blood also carries and supplies nutrients (absorbed from the digestive system) and hormones. It removes waste products from cells and these are then detoxified primarily by the liver and kidneys (and the lungs in the case of carbon dioxide). The blood is also involved in regulating the body's pH (acidity or alkalinity) levels, water content and temperature. In addition, constituents carried in the blood enable clotting to prevent blood loss when we are cut or damaged, and the body's defences are maintained through the activity of the immune system.

The heart receives blood depleted of oxygen from the veins and it pumps this into the lungs for re-oxygenation. The revitalised blood returns to the heart, from where it is pumped out into the general cir-culation. Blood courses through the arteries and is delivered to the body's cells through thin capillaries. These capillaries allow the movement of oxygen-rich arterial blood into the tissues at one end and carbon dioxide-rich blood into the capillaries at the other. From there, the capillaries connect to the veins. The heart pumps blood out through the arteries but the return of blood to the heart through the veins is mainly achieved through pumping of the blood upwards by the action of our muscles as we walk, run and stretch. The major difference between the arteries and the veins is that the latter contain valves at regular intervals to prevent backflow of blood as it moves up towards the heart. The arteries, by contrast, are simple, hollow muscular tubes.

# Blood and the emotions

There are a number of words that we use to describe the blood and these describe our conception of its functions or powers as being beyond the merely physical. We talk of there being 'bad blood' between warring parties, or of an impetuous person being 'hot blooded'. When we are angry about something we say that our 'blood boils', and if we are afraid we might feel that our 'blood runs cold'. If speaking of an uncaring or weak person we might say that they are 'bloodless'.

As with the blood we have many commonplace ways of describing the heart. When we are sad we say we have a 'heavy heart'; by contrast, when we are happy we have a sensation of feeling 'light-hearted'. We consider the heart to be an emotional organ, unlike the brain, and when we are in a quandary over a difficult decision we might say that 'my heart says "yes" but my brain says "no".' We draw a distinction between the intuitive, feeling nature of the heart and the rational, objective nature of the brain. The heart is a symbol of love and caring. Our perception of the heart as an emotional force is such that we can say someone died of a 'broken heart'.

These emotional associations with the heart and the blood are understandable because it is noticeable how our heart responds when we experience strong feelings. The rate and rhythm of the heart alter as we experience anxiety, fear, shock, sexual arousal, joy and peace. These changes are brought about by the effects of our autonomic nervous system on our cardiovascular activity. The autonomic nervous system communicates signals from the brain to the heart and blood vessels in response to changes in the physical and emotional environment. This also meets the needs of the body as we move between different levels of physical activity – when we exert ourselves the heart has to pump harder and faster; when we relax the heart can slow down and relax.

This connection between the state of our cardiovascular system and our mental and emotional state is important because it means that what we think and what we feel can have a direct impact on how our heart and blood vessels behave. The negative effects of stress in a challenging world can adversely affect our heart and this 'uptight' state is one of the major contributing causes of an increase in high blood pressure.

## Nurturing a Healthy Heart

There are several things that we can do in order to promote a healthy cardiovascular system and help prevent future heart disease. Amongst the most important of these are:

- Maintaining a healthy blood pressure;
- Controlling cholesterol levels;
- Reducing our risk of late-onset diabetes.

### Blood pressure

We can live with high blood pressure for a long time without feeling unwell in any way. One of the major difficulties with this condition is that we do not experience ill effects until the problem is firmly established. When the ill effects do finally manifest they can be very severe. The most serious potential consequences are heart failure or stroke (a bleed into the brain). Because high blood pressure can remain hidden for a long time without being discovered, it is important to ensure that our blood pressure is kept within a healthy range. All adults should have their blood pressure taken regularly – at least once or twice a year. The normal range of blood pressure varies depending on sex, age and activity, but an ideal figure is usually around 120 over 80 (blood pressure is measured in millimetres of mercury, abbreviated to mmHg). The higher figure is called the systolic blood pressure and the lower one is the diastolic blood pressure. When you have your blood pressure taken, an inflatable cuff is placed around your arm and this obstructs the blood flow through the arm as it is pumped up. As air is let out, the level of pressure at which the sound or pulsations of the returning circulation start to appear is called the systolic pressure; the point where those impulses cease as the circulation in the arm returns to normal is called the diastolic blood pressure. The risk of cardiovascular disease increases significantly when our diastolic blood pressure rises consistently above 90–95 – ideally, it should stay below 90. Doctors will normally begin a course of treatment if the diastolic figure rises above 100.

## Cholesterol

High cholesterol levels can have a major impact on cardiovascular health. As cholesterol accumulates along the walls of blood vessels it narrows them and can eventually block them, cutting off the blood supply to the areas that the artery serves. The tissues in that area can consequently become damaged and cease to function normally – if indeed at all. Clearly, this is a particular problem if it occurs in the coronary arteries that service the heart itself. A combination of high blood pressure and high cholesterol is a serious cause for concern as they carry an even greater risk when found together.

Not all cholesterol is unhealthy. The body has the ability to manufacture its own cholesterol because there are several essential bodily functions for which it is required. Cholesterol is used to make bile, which is used to aid the absorption of fats from the digestive system. Cholesterol is also used as a building block in making steroid hormones, including the sex hormones oestrogen, progesterone and testosterone, and as part of the protective outer layer of the skin – cholesterol helps form the corneum, the waxy layer covering the skin that helps prevent excessive evaporation of water from the body and stops harmful substances from passing across the skin barrier into the body. However, its main function is in forming the fatty membranes of all the body's cells. Cholesterol when in balance is a natural and essential substance; the problem lies in having too much of it – and too much of the wrong kind of cholesterol.

There are two types of cholesterol – LDL (low-density lipoprotein) cholesterol and HDL (high-density lipoprotein) cholesterol. LDL cholesterol is often described as 'bad' cholesterol because in excess it can cause adverse effects. HDL cholesterol is known as 'good' cholesterol because it gives us all the beneficial effects of cholesterol and none of the bad effects. In fact, having a high level of HDL cholesterol in proportion to LDL cholesterol means that we carry a significantly decreased risk of developing heart disease. The dietary advice given below can assist in ensuring that your cholesterol levels are kept in balance.

## Diabetes

We are not concerned here with early-onset insulin-dependent diabetes (Type 1 diabetes), although it is of course a significant health problem, but with late-onset (occurring in adulthood – usually over 40 years of age) non-insulin-dependent diabetes (Type 2 diabetes). Late onset diabetes is a condition that is becoming increasing common, and it contributes strongly to cardiovascular illness. It is also largely preventable.

Late-onset diabetes does not occur because we have a deficiency of insulin (the hormone we use to metabolise glucose), but because our cells become resistant to the effects of insulin. This happens when we have a diet that is too rich in carbohydrates (sugar-rich foods). Our bodies become saturated with sugar and, because the cells can no longer use it all, they start to resist the demands of insulin to let sugar in. This means that taking insulin, as with Type 1 diabetes, is not an effective treatment. This is called Insulin Resistance Syndrome, also known as Syndrome X, and it leads to late-onset diabetes. It has been estimated that at least 66 million people worldwide currently suffer from Syndrome X. The vast majority of sufferers are in the West because Syndrome X is a condition of affluent, overfed societies. It can be difficult to diagnose Syndrome X because, although it leads to late-onset diabetes, it will not necessarily feature high glucose levels in the sugar or blood (the main ways of detecting diabetes) until the illness has actually developed. However, if you are currently overweight, eat a carbohydrate rich diet, and crave sugary foods, it is possible that you have

Syndrome X and you would be advised to take action before late-onset diabetes sets in.

The problem with late-onset diabetes is that when the body is unable to metabolise sugar, it stores it as fat (triglycerides) and this can cause the same kind of problems for the heart and blood vessels as cholesterol. These fats can also damage the fine blood vessels (micro-vasculature) in the body, leading to damage to the eyes, kidneys and nerves. The key factors in beating Syndrome X are to:

- Maintain a diet low in high-glycaemic index foods (sugar-rich foods that release sugar into the bloodstream very quickly);
- Keep a healthy weight (lose weight if you are obese);
- Follow a regular exercise programme.

A number of herbs can be excellent for treating Syndrome X: see the section on herbs for the cardiovascular system beginning on page 159. (*See* page 253 for my Syndrome X diet advice sheet which I give to my patients. This advice is easy to follow and many patients have had very good results from working with it.)

## Looking After Your Diet

Given the large number of people affected by heart disease, it is unsurprising that many products are sold with the promise that they are 'high in fibre', 'rich in antioxidants' or 'low in cholesterol – virtually fat free'. Unfortunately, it is often the case that these products do not contain the best types of fibre, antioxidants or fats. When manufacturers label their products with such health claims, they may qualify them by saying that their high-fibre product can help prevent heart disease 'as part of a controlled diet'. Sometimes it is difficult to decide what to do for the best, but quite a lot is now known about which dietary changes will help us care for our hearts and blood vessels.

A study into why the incidence of heart disease in many Mediterranean countries seems to be lower than that in other developed countries found that the diet in this region tended to have a number of features that protected the heart and circulation from damage; these can be summarised as:

- High in fibre;
- Low in saturated fat and high in monounsaturated and polyunsaturated fats (such as olive oil);
- Rich in fruit and vegetables (the consumption of another source of antioxidants, red wine, may also help us attain better cardiovascular health).

By contrast, many other countries in the West have a national diet that is low in fibre, high in saturated fat and low in fruit and vegetables. The evidence from studies such as this makes it possible to give good specific advice about what constitutes the essentials of a good cardiovascular diet.

## Low salt

Around a third of the general population in the West has an inherited genetic sensitivity to salt. If you are a member of this third – and if you have high blood pressure, it is likely that you are – you should avoid salt completely. Even if you do not have high blood pressure it is wise to keep salt intake to a minimum – too much salt can cause ill effects (including increasing the removal of calcium from the body, perhaps contributing to the development of osteo-porosis) even in people who are not salt sensitive.

Convenience foods tend to be high in salt and should be avoided. Try instead to cook with individual natural fresh ingredients and avoid adding salt to food, so that you can cultivate your palate to appreciate natural subtle flavours. Also, be wary of manufacturers' attempts to disguise the salt content in their products by referring to it as sodium instead of salt.

## High in soluble fibre

Fibre can absorb excess cholesterol from the bowel, helping to remove it from the body. The best type of fibre is soluble fibre from fruit, vegetables and whole grains – other types of fibre may be irritants to the bowel. A diet with a high intake of fruit and vegetables, eaten with their skins left on where appropriate, and a variety of grains should supply all the soluble fibre we need.

## Low in sugar

Avoid simple (quickly released) carbohydrates, such as sugar, as the body can convert these to fat; eat instead complex (slow release) carbohydrates, such as whole grains instead.

## High in antioxidants

Regular antioxidant intake helps to reduce the risk of heart disease (*see* chapter 5).

## Low in saturated fat and high in monounsaturated and polyunsaturated fats

Fats come in different forms, some of which are good for us while others can be very harmful. The more saturated a fat is (the more hydrogen molecules it has attached to it) the more harmful it is. As a rule, any fat that sets hard at room temperature, such as animal fats, lard, butter and margarine, are likely to be bad for us, and any oils that remain runny are likely to be OK. Fats that set hard outside the body set hard inside the body; runny fats (by and large) do not.

### Butter and margarine

While many margarines are made from runny oils they tend to have hydrogen added to them to turn them into saturated fats. Therefore, one should avoid 'hydrogenated' margarines. In addition, the chemical manipulation involved in turning runny fats into solid fats means that many margarines contain 'trans-fatty acids', which can be carcinogenic. So, advocates of butter have some good arguments against margarine; however, butter remains a saturated fat and is not a healthy food to eat. It is best to try to avoid both margarine and butter as far as possible. Olive oil spread on bread as an alternative takes a little getting used to but can work very well.

## Oils

We should regularly consume unsaturated fats such as olive oil (high in monounsaturated fatty acids) and sunflower oil (high in polyunsaturated fatty acids); these healthy oils should not be heated but taken added to spreads, dips and salad dressings. Frying oils generally should be avoided as this decreases their positive qualities and generates trans-fatty acids; it is better to grill foods lightly instead (grilling till charred generates dioxins which are also carcinogenic).

## Essential fatty acids (EFAs)

Included in the mono- and polyunsaturated fatty acids group are the essential fatty acids (EFAs). EFAs have excellent health benefits for the cardiovascular and other bodily systems, particularly the omega-6 and omega-3 EFAs. They are used, like cholesterol, to form the membranes of the body's cells. The membranes formed from EFAs are flexible and resilient, and are capable of functioning more effectively than those formed from saturated fats. The body will make cell membranes from the fats that are available to it – taking EFAs will enable the body to produce healthier cells that improve overall health and are more resistant to disease. This means that it is beneficial to eat a healthy balance of the omega-6 and omega-3 EFAs, ideally at a ratio of 4:1 (4 times as much omega-6 as omega-3). We tend to consume too much omega-6 and too little omega-3, so it is a good idea to take a general supplement such as flax oil (also known as linseed oil) or hemp oil – about 1 teaspoon a day of either oil should be taken.

Fish oils also have protective effects for the heart. It is a good idea to eat oily fish (such as sardines, herring and mackerel) 2–3 times a week.

## Moderate alcohol intake

Red wine may be of some value in providing a source of cardioprotective antioxidants. If you wish to drink red wine as part of a Mediterranean diet approach, avoid binge drinking but have up to 2–3 glasses of red wine a day, taken with meals. Drink a glass of water for every glass of wine consumed. It is wise to have 2 days a week that are completely alcohol free.

## Avoid caffeine

Caffeine can stress the heart and constrict the blood vessels, thereby exacerbating high blood pressure. In addition, caffeine affects sugar metabolism and can add to problems with Syndrome X (*see* page 151). Coffee and fizzy drinks containing caffeine are best avoided – learn to enjoy alternatives such as barley and rye drinks, dandelion coffee and herbal teas instead.

## No smoking

In addition to its better-known carcinogenic effects, smoking also enhances the ability of cholesterol to stick to the walls of blood vessels. If you smoke you really need to consider giving up – being a non-smoker is a fundamental health attribute. Psychology, hypnotherapy, acupuncture and herbal medicine can all assist in the process of stopping smoking.

# Lifestyle Improvements

While diet is crucial in helping us to attain optimum cardiovascular health there are several other areas that we can work on.

## Stress management

The demands of modern life, the high cost of living, the insecurity of the job market, the need for both partners in a relationship to work (even when there are children), and the lack of an extended family or other close support network can all contribute to stress.

Because we often feel that the many demands on us are out of our control, this may lead to feelings of depression and the inability to cope. When stress reaches this level it can have a physical as well as psychological impact on us.

Mental and emotional stress exacerbates high blood pressure, increasing the load on the cardiovascular system. It is important to try and reduce the sources of stress and take steps to lessen its effects. Looking at alternative ways of living our lives and earning our incomes, retraining for a better career, and building up a support network with similarly pressured friends can be of great benefit.

Learn to prioritise your work and manage your time so that you complete your tasks as effectively as possible, leaving you with space to relax and 'destress' (see page 158 for advice on relaxation).

## Maintain an ideal weight

It is important to avoid becoming obese and to reduce your weight if you already are overweight. Being overweight significantly increases the risk of developing late-onset diabetes and heart disease. Some people find it easier to maintain a healthy weight than others, but there are only two proven ways of effectively keeping a good weight or reducing excessive weight and these are diet and exercise. Adopting the Syndrome X diet will help on the diet front (see page 253). If you need help in dealing with your weight, discuss the matter with your doctor, herbalist or nutritionist.

## Exercise

Regular exercise is essential for your health in general and for a healthy cardiovascular system in particular. Exercise helps the return of blood to the heart through the veins and will help prevent the development of varicose veins. It also improves the efficiency and tone of the heart and blood vessels, burns up sugar and fats that might otherwise coat the arteries, and reduces weight. It is important that exercise is regular and that you choose a form of exercise that you enjoy.

Walking, swimming and cycling are all excellent forms of exercise. Taking part in a sport such as football, tennis or basketball is also very beneficial but you should be careful not to work on one part of the body too much at the expense of the others as this can lead to strains and injuries. Aggressive sports such as squash may not be the best exercise for everyone – long periods of inactivity interspersed with short, sharp bursts of intense exercise can be stressful for the body. Moderate, balanced regular exercise is to be preferred. Working out in a gym can be very good exercise but if you are new to that kind of exercise you should discuss your needs with a qualified instructor before you begin. Running can also be good exercise and many people take up jogging in order to improve their fitness. However, running on hard ground (such as pavements) can lead to knee and spine problems, so it is best to run on soft ground only (grassy areas).

## Relaxation

It is as important to relax as it is to exercise; the two should be balanced. People often associate relaxing with sitting and doing nothing in particular, but there is a distinction to be made between relaxation and resting. Resting is a passive state of inactivity and sleep is the most important form of rest that we all experience. It sounds like a contradiction in terms but we need to involve ourselves actively in achieving relaxation. This means that just as we might decide to take up swimming as a form of exercise, we need to consider which activities we can take up as a form of relaxation. We can specifically seek to become relaxed rather than relying on relaxation just happening to us when we stop doing things. Relaxation can occur at the physical, emotional or mental level – and sometimes on all three at once.

Excellent types of relaxation include meditation, yoga, tai chi, having a luxurious warm bath, receiving a massage, listening to calming music, spending a quiet evening in gentle conversation with friends, spending time watching and listening to the sea, or contemplating a favourite view or location.

# Herbs for the Cardiovascular System

Herbs can be of great value in improving cardiovascular function and preventing disease. Antioxidant herbs (*see* Chapter 6) are some of the major protective herbs for the heart. Beyond this, herbs can assist in lowering blood pressure, lowering cholesterol, and improving the performance of the heart and the tone of the blood vessels.

In traditional herbal medicine, herbs that can stimulate the circulation and enhance heat in the body, such as chilli peppers (*Capsicum* species), ginger (*Zingiber officinalis*) and horseradish (*Armoracia rusticana*), have long been prized. The traditional herbal approach to acute severe disease, especially infectious disease, has been to use diaphoretic herbs (inducing sweating) and circulatory stimulants in combination to raise the vital energies of the body to throw off the condition. Such herbs can:

- Improve the blood supply to the heart;
- Stimulate the heart muscles to beat faster and stronger;
- Increase the muscular contractions of blood vessels;
- Dilate the blood vessels so that blood can pass more freely through them.

**Keeping warm** – Some of the stronger stimulant herbs, such as chilli peppers, can be unsuitable for people who have high blood pressure or a weakness of the heart. Herbs in this category can be useful for people who suffer from low blood pressure or who are prone to having cold hands and feet, finding it hard to keep warm.

**Mental stimulants** – Several circulatory stimulant herbs have a particular affinity for improving blood flow to the brain: gingko (*Gingko biloba*) is particularly famous for this, while rosemary (*Rosmarinus officinalis*) has long been famed for improving mental performance and memory. Interest is currently reviving in lesser periwinkle (*Vinca minor*), which is referred to in several old herbal texts as having profound effects on enhancing mental activities.

159

**Relaxants** – While circulatory stimulants can be very useful for those, especially older people, who have normal or low blood pressure, many people experience more benefit from using herbs that relax the heart and blood vessels, helping to slow the heart rate and lower the blood pressure, easing the tension in the cardiovascular system. Herbs that have these properties include valerian (*Valeriana officinalis*) and lemon balm (*Melissa officinalis*) (*see* chapter 14). These herbs act on the brain and central nervous system to cause a general relaxation in the body, including the heart. Valerian has proven to be very useful in treating states of anxiety that lead to cardiovascular symptoms such as palpitations (awareness of the heart beating in a fast or irregular manner). The aptly named cramp bark (*Viburnum opulus*) relaxes tension in the blood vessels and can help reduce high blood pressure, as can limeflowers (*Tilia* species), which make a very pleasant tea for regular use to calm tension in the cardiovascular system. Motherwort (*Leonurus cardiaca*) is often of value in reducing high blood pressure and is thought of as a mild sedative for the heart.

**Lowering the cholesterol** – A number of herbs have been shown to aid the lowering of cholesterol levels in conjunction with dietary changes; these include garlic (*Allium sativum*) and fenugreek (*Trigonella foenum-graecum*). The Masai tribe in East Africa have an extremely high-cholesterol diet, subsisting as they do primarily on the meat, milk and blood of their cattle. Scientists have discovered that the Masai protect themselves from the harmful effects of long-term high-cholesterol exposure by adding the bark of the East Indian walnut (*Albizia lebbeck*) to the pot when they are cooking.

**Syndrome X and late-onset diabetes** – Several herbs help to tackle Syndrome X and late-onset diabetes, including goat's rue (*Galega officinalis*) and the Ayurvedic herb gurmar (*Gymnema sylvestre*). Gurmar is a fascinating herb: its name translates as 'sugar destroyer' and it can actually reduce sugar cravings, so making it easier to give up eating sweet foods. It also lowers blood sugar levels and cholesterol.

**Improving the tone of blood vessels** – Rutin is a constituent of several herbs, including buckwheat (*Fagopyrum esculentum*), and it helps to reduce fragility in the capillaries making them less likely to rupture and bleed. Taking this herb as a food or as a rutin supplement can be particularly relevant if you are getting older and starting to notice that you bruise easily (this can be a common benign disorder but may also suggest more serious disease so see your doctor or herbalist before trying rutin). It can also be of use if you suffer from chilblains. A cream made from conkers, the seeds of the horse chestnut (*Aesculus hippocastanum*), can help to relieve symptoms of heavy or tired legs, and reduce the prominence of vessels in the legs if you suffer from varicose veins.

*Caution*
Below are given the profiles of several herbs that you might want to consider taking to assist your cardiovascular system, but before doing so there is a word of caution. If you have high blood pressure there are some herbs that will not be suitable for you. If you are in any doubt, consult a herbalist.

As a general rule, if you are taking any kind of medication for problems in this area, talk to your doctor and a herbalist before taking herbs for the heart and circulation. Never take cardio-vascular herbs without the specific advice of an experienced herbal practitioner. Obtain the express approval of your doctor if you are taking any kind of blood-thinning drugs (anticoagulants such as warfarin and heparin) or heart-stimulant drugs, especially digoxin and digitoxin.

The herbs described below could become your trusted supporters in achieving and sustaining a healthy heart and circulation.

## Cramp bark

This plant is a European shrub also known as Guelder rose (*Viburnum opulus*). The bark scraped from the thin stems is used in

herbal medicine. The effect of the herb is to open up the arteries
by relaxing them and relieving tension in the circulation. It is a
useful herb to take as a tea if you have borderline or mildly raised
blood pressure, and it mixes well with cinnamon bark, which
offsets the natural bitterness of cramp bark and adds a warming
element which complements the relaxant effects of cramp bark.
Use 1 teaspoon of cramp bark and 1 teaspoon of cinnamon bark
per cup and drink 2–3 cups of per day made by decoction.

## Fenugreek

Fenugreek (*Trigonella foenum-graecum*) is best known as a
constituent of curries but it also has important medicinal
qualities because it lowers blood sugar and cholesterol levels. If
you have Syndrome X, taking this herb while following the diet
plan (*see* page 253) can be very beneficial. It is best taken as a
powder (drunk in a glass of water) with the average adult dose
being 1 level dessertspoon per day taken in the morning with
breakfast. This may not sound like a pleasant idea but you will
get used to it, especially when you see the results it has for your
health.

Fenugreek has a stimulant effect on the liver and some people
notice that they experience looseness of the bowels and
increased perspiration or sweating on commencing taking it.
Don't worry – this is a natural detoxification process. Some
people also experience that they smell of curry for a while after
taking it. These reactions usually settle down after 1–2 weeks of
taking fenugreek. If they do not, try lowering the dose by degrees
until these mild side effects disappear.

## Garlic

A folk saying has it that 'garlic is as good as ten mothers'. It is
certainly true that garlic (*Allium sativum*) is one of the most

important herbs for the heart and circulation, and this is why I have chosen it as the key herb for the cardiovascular system (*see* page 167). Garlic is a fine example of a plant that acts as both a food and a medicine; it is very safe and effective in both respects. Garlic reduces the levels of cholesterol and triglycerides in the blood. It also lowers blood pressure and inhibits the effects of platelets (blood-clotting agents) thereby having anticoagulant activity. This means that garlic is excellent for protecting the arteries from becoming blocked, helping to ensure that the blood supply is adequately maintained through the body, particularly in the coronary arteries supplying the heart. However, the anticoagulant power of garlic is so potent that you should consider not taking it if you are already taking anticoagulants, and it should be avoided before undergoing surgery because it may impair the normal blood-clotting response.

Other close members of the garlic family can also have positive effects in caring for the heart and these include onions (*Allium cepa*), leeks (*Allium ampeloprasum*), chives (*Allium schoenoprasum*), and wild garlic or ransoms (*Allium ursinum*).

## Ginger

As well as being a very popular culinary item, ginger (*Zingiber officinale*) has long been used for its medicinal properties, which are wide ranging. With regards to the cardiovascular system, they include improving circulation to the limbs, and anticoagulant activity that reduces the formation of blockages in the arteries. Ginger is a worthwhile item to include regularly as a flavouring in the diet either in fresh or dried form. Combined with slices of fresh garlic and lemon, it makes an excellent refreshing and warming tea with antioxidant and circulatory stimulant properties. Ginger is not so strong in its action that you need to be concerned if you have high blood pressure, but its circulatory strengthening effect is nonetheless strong enough to be worthwhile.

## Gingko

Ginkgo (*Gingko biloba*) is one of the best-selling herbal products and will be familiar to many. It improves blood flow, especially to the brain and legs, facilitating enhanced oxygen and nutrition supplies to these areas. It is an excellent antioxidant and improves memory and mental activity. This herb is particularly useful for older people to inhibit age-related changes in mental faculties, and it can be taken on a daily basis for long periods of time. It is a good herb to take at times of increased demand on mental performance such as during revision for examinations or when preparing a major project or presentation. If you are constantly using your brain creatively and have regularly to perform prolonged feats of intensive concentration, this herb may be one that will benefit you if taken on a regular basis.

Gingko may also be of help if you experience dizziness (always check out this symptom with your doctor or herbalist), tinnitus or headaches. It also has a role in treating and preventing diseases of the eye such as macular degeneration, and in slowing down the progression of Alzheimer's disease. Take gingko leaf as a tea made by infusion: use 2–3 teaspoons per cup and take 2–3 cups a day for general enhancing and preventive cardiovascular purposes. It tastes quite pleasant and can be combined with other cardiovascular herbs such as hawthorn.

## Hawthorn

Hawthorn (*Crataegus* species) was discussed earlier with regard to its antioxidant properties (*see* page 91) – these help protect against cardiovascular disease but there is more to hawthorn's role in caring for the heart. It improves blood flow through the coronary arteries, thereby improving oxygen and nutrient supply to the heart muscle, and it improves the force of heart contractions and helps normalise the rhythm of the heartbeat.

In addition, it reduces high blood pressure. The combination of these actions means that it is an excellent herbal medicine for you to use if you have a family history of conditions such as angina, high blood pressure, cholesterol problems, heart failure, strokes or heart attacks. It is also a very safe herb to take.

Take hawthorn leaves and flowers as a tea made by infusion. Use 2 teaspoons per cup and take 2–3 cups each day. Hawthorn tea has a pleasant taste and can be used safely on a regular long-term basis. If you suffer from low blood pressure or from postural hypotension (where you experience a transient dizziness with changes of posture such as bending over or standing up), hawthorn is best avoided as it could potentially lower your blood pressure still further. If you are going through periods of stress where you are experiencing feelings of tension you can take hawthorn mixed with lemon balm or limeflowers.

## Olive

Olive oil has already been mentioned as a good source of healthy monounsaturated fats (see page 155). Olive trees (Olea europea) are long-lived, beautiful plants that are a crucial element in the Mediterranean diet. The oil promotes an increase in healthy HDL cholesterol and a decrease in harmful LDL cholesterol and also helps reduce blood pressure. In professional herbal medicine, the leaves are prescribed as a tea or tincture in addition to the oil.

It is a good idea to take olive oil and garlic together to gain the benefits of both. One way of doing this is to crush 1 clove of garlic and mix it with 2 teaspoons of olive oil. This garlic oil can then be spread on wholemeal bread in place of butter or margarine, topped with salad and eaten.

# Rosemary

Rosemary (*Rosmarinus officinalis*), originating from the Mediterranean, is a herb full of sunshine and scent. It contains the potent antioxidant carnosic acid. Rosemary has a longstanding reputation as a herb that improves the memory, attested to by the saying that 'rosemary is for remembrance'. It is generally warming to the circulation and can be an excellent herb to take if you suffer from cold hands and feet, or feel that your circulation is sluggish or poor. It can also prove useful if you suffer from low blood pressure. Although rosemary is not so strongly stimulating that it will cause agitation, it should nevertheless be avoided in the evenings as it can interfere with sleep by keeping the brain active and wakeful.

Rosemary should be used regularly in the kitchen, added to soups, stews, sauces and other foods. It is a good idea to grow rosemary and add it fresh, chopped fine, to salads and sandwiches. Rosemary tea can be a good way of taking this plant, but it is not to everybody's taste. If you do enjoy it, use 1 teaspoon of dried rosemary or 3 teaspoons of fresh per cup, infuse for 10 minutes (keeping the pot or cup covered to retain the volatile oils) and take a cup twice daily. If you wish to harness the benefits of rosemary but do not like the tea then you can take a dose of the tincture. Take 3–6ml per day of the 1:2 tincture.

# GARLIC

**Scientific name** *Allium sativum*

**Plant family** Liliaceae

**Type of plant** Bulb.

**Part used** Cloves from the bulb.

**Phytochemicals** Depends on the type of preparation. Dried garlic contains alliin and alliinase. Crushed fresh garlic contains alliicin. Alliin and alliicin are compounds that contain sulphur.

**Actions** Antithrombotic; hypocholesterolaemic; hypotensive.

**Indications** High cholesterol levels, high blood pressure. As a general dietary aid to prevent heart disease.

**Preparations** Capsules of dried garlic powder; fermented 'odourless' garlic; garlic oil; fresh cloves. I prefer to recommend the fresh clove although research evidence exists to support the use of other types of preparation as well. Take 1–2 cloves of fresh garlic each day crushed and spread on a sandwich or in salad dressing.

**Combinations** With fresh garlic there can be a concern about the smell of garlic on the breath. This usually decreases with regular use, but can be reduced to some extent by taking garlic with aromatic herbs such as parsley and coriander, which will mask the smell.

**Cautions** Do not take raw garlic on its own; this can cause burning of the mouth and irritation to the digestive system. Raw garlic may sometimes exacerbate heartburn (reflux oesophagitis). Only take garlic alongside anticoagulant drugs on the advice of your doctor. Avoid taking garlic for 10 days before undergoing a surgical operation.

**Conservation** Garlic is widely cultivated for dietary and medicinal use.

# Chapter 11

# HERBS FOR THE RESPIRATORY SYSTEM –

## 'The breath of life'

There is an inseparable relationship between the respiratory system and the circulation, between the blood and the air. The vital function of the respiratory system is to take oxygen into the body and to expel carbon dioxide out of the body; it is the job of the circulation to absorb oxygen from the lungs and to transport it around the body, as well as bringing carbon dioxide to the lungs to be exhaled.

## The Respiratory System

The respiratory system can be divided into upper and lower parts. The main structures in the upper respiratory tract are the nose and mouth (through which we move air in and out of the body), and the throat (or pharynx). In the lower respiratory tract the pharynx connects to the larynx (or voice box) and trachea, which combine to form a tube that connects with the lungs. A number of structures are associated with the respiratory system, including the nasal sinuses, the ears (which are connected to the sinuses by the Eustachian or auditory tube), and the lymph glands in the head and neck.

### The lungs

The structure of the lungs is sometimes compared to an upended tree with the trachea (the main airway connecting the mouth and nose with lungs) as the tree trunk and the tubes leading off the trachea (the bronchi) as branches. In fact, these are known technically as the 'branches of the bronchial tree'. At the end of the bronchi are the fine membranes (alveoli) that allow oxygen and carbon dioxide to pass across them between the blood and the air.

The lungs have an extraordinary capacity for gaseous exchange. The alveoli are so thin that our lungs can contain up to 30 million of them – if they were laid out flat they could cover an area the size of a tennis court. Just as our heart beats automatically, so we breathe in and out automatically, the rate at which we breathe depending on the level of our physical activity. Our breathing rate is controlled by the respiratory centre in the brain.

## Mucus

Since air, particularly warm air, is drying, and because the air that we breathe may contain particles that we do not want to take into our lungs, such as dust, smoke and pollution, the body has developed strategies to prevent the lungs from drying out and becoming clogged with unwanted matter. A layer of mucus coats the lining of the respiratory system to keep the airways lubricated and to trap foreign matter. However, an excess of this mucus can cause congestion, while a deficiency can leave one at risk of developing inflammation and infection, so this needs to be kept in balance. The respiratory tract is lined with tiny, hair-like protuberances called cilia, which move together in waves to shift the mucus up out of the lungs, either to be swallowed (and then destroyed in the stomach by its high acid levels) or to be coughed up and spat out (expectorated). This mechanism is known as the mucociliary escalator.

## Common Respiratory Problems

A large number of medical conditions can arise in the respiratory system, ranging from mild to severe disorders. Some of the most common are:

- Asthma,
- Chest infections (such as pneumonia and tuberculosis),
- Coughs and colds,
- Hay fever,
- Lung cancer,
- Middle ear disease (otitis media or glue ear),
- Sinusitis,
- Sore throat.

We all experience coughs and colds from time to time but a weakened immune system will mean that we develop them more frequently. Asthma is a very common problem today with the number of people suffering from this condition on the increase. Lung cancer remains the most widespread form of cancer in the West. In some ways, the prevalence of respiratory disease reflects the vulnerability of this system – the respiratory tract is literally open to the outside world. We cannot close ourselves off from the atmosphere in which we live; we must constantly breathe it in, whatever it is carrying.

## Environmental Pollution

Environmental pollution is one of the major causes of respiratory disease. Some of this might be considered natural pollution by allergens, such as pollen and household dust, that cause seasonal rhinitis (hay fever) and perennial rhinitis (a type of hay fever reaction that persists all year round). The most important man-made pollution is that generated by burning fossil fuels in power stations, industry and cars. Tobacco smoke is either a pollutant that is self-inflicted by smokers, or a true environmental pollutant for non-smokers exposed to tobacco fumes (passive smokers).

## Inhalers

Of increasing concern is the practice of prescribing inhalers, given by doctors to relieve difficulty in breathing. Inhalers can play a crucial role in the treatment of asthma, but this is a diagnosis that can be arrived at too readily. People who just have a cough and cold, who may be experiencing a reaction to pollution or who have a temporary chest infection are frequently diagnosed as having asthma and given inhalers. Sometimes, when a correct diagnosis is made, they may be given inhalers anyway to help them breathe 'until things settle down'. The lungs can quickly become habituated to inhalers and many people find it hard to stop using them.

## Looking after the Respiratory System

Faced with exposure to high levels of pollution and with our vulnerable lungs protected by little more than a thin layer of mucus, it helps to optimise the resilience of the respiratory system. The three major areas to look at here are diet, exercise and environmental pollution.

### Diet

Many people experience difficulties in producing mucus of the right quality or quantity. Catarrh (excessive production of thick mucus) can cause congestion and play a role in chronic sinus problems, chest infections and fatigue (by impairing natural breathing and limiting exercise). Catarrh can be something that occurs by itself, but it also plays an important part in several respiratory diseases, especially asthma. If suffering with catarrh, including in asthma and chronic sinusitis, it is important to follow a diet that reduces solid mucus formation and promotes the movement of mucus. The most significant mucus-forming foods are dairy products. In particular, milk and cheese tend to stimulate unhealthy mucus formation that is static, solid and hard to dislodge. Many of my catarrhal patients only begin to improve when they completely avoid dairy products.

Our early hunter-gatherer ancestors would not have eaten dairy products and in many Asian countries dairy products are still rarely or never consumed. In the West, the importance of dairy products in promoting healthy bones has been overemphasised and many of us have grown up being given free milk at school. Interestingly, at present there are plans to give free fruit to students in schools in the UK. Research suggests that this will bring far more benefits than free milk. Bones are made up of a number of minerals, including magnesium and boron in addition to calcium. The key nutrient that we need to consume in proportion to calcium is magnesium in an optimum ratio of 2:1. Plant sources of calcium such as nuts, seeds, grains, pulses and vegetables contain calcium in this ideal ratio. For cows milk, however, the ratio is 11:1 and for cheese it is 22:1.

Other cold, mucus-forming foods include white flour products (such as cakes, pastries and bread), sugary foods, bananas and peanut butter. If you have problems with catarrh you should avoid these foods, as well as dairy products. Also, ensure you eat plenty of foods that help to thin and loosen mucus. Such foods include:

- Fruit and vegetables in general,
- Simple root vegetable soups,
- Raw fruit and vegetable salads,
- Garlic and onions,
- Warming culinary herbs and spices such as chilli, cinnamon and cloves.

Antioxidants are particularly important in the diet for their role in helping to prevent cancer, especially since lung cancer is the most prevalent of all cancers in the West. Antioxidants can also be of value in helping to prevent or treat a number of other chest conditions, including asthma.

## Exercise

During exercise, our breathing rate increases and we use our lungs to their full capacity. This provides exercise for the muscles and tissues of the respiratory system, improving their tone and general functioning. Exercise also promotes the clearance of mucus and stimulates the blood supply to the lungs, thereby enhancing respiratory performance overall.

Breathing exercises can also help treat chest problems such as asthma. A useful exercise is to focus on the breath while meditating.

*Breathing Exercise*

- Sit comfortably in a warm environment where you will not be disturbed.
- Close your eyes and begin to become aware of your breathing.
- After a little while, start to focus on breathing in positive things with each inspiration (peace, relaxation, joy, love – whatever suits you) and breathing out negative things with each expiration (anger, tension, irritation – whatever concerns you).
- Do this for 5–10 minutes or until you feel a sense of completion, then slowly open your eyes and return to your environment.

## Pollution

It is the nature of pollution that it blows around the whole world. Some places are more pure than others, but very few are completely free of the effects of pollution. We now know that asthma, as well as being associated with a genetic predisposition, can be made worse by fossil fuel pollution. The closer you live to a busy main road the more likely you are to develop asthma.

A new house in an unspoilt area is not available to all of us, but we can try to control the environment within our own homes and, to some extent, in our workplaces. It is necessary for all of us to keep our exposure to pollutants to a minimum. The following are some useful guidelines:

- Do not smoke and try not to breathe in other people's tobacco smoke.
- Avoid strongly scented household cleaning products and cosmetics. Artificial scents of the kind used in washing-up liquids, soap powders and deodorants can be extremely aggressive and even carcinogenic. Instead, choose gentle, hypoallergenic (meaning that it is unlikely to cause an allergic reaction), environmentally friendly products.

- Be careful when buying household items such as sofas and carpets. They may have been sprayed with antifungal and flame-retardant chemicals that can be unhealthy in other ways. Try and find alternatives to these products or put new purchases in isolation with the windows open to air out for a few days before starting to live with them.

- Remember, in addition to causing problems with cholesterol, fried foods can generate toxic fumes, so make sure that your kitchen is well ventilated.

- Dust in general, and the house dust mite in particular, can exacerbate asthma, sinusitis and allergic rhinitis. To minimise the effects it is a good idea to try and keep carpets to a minimum, having wooden floors with rugs instead.

- When vacuuming, use a machine that has a good filter so that dust is not recirculated into the air.

- An effective way of inhibiting a build-up of dust mites in bedding is to place duvets and pillows in a chest freezer for 24 hours, once a week – this will kill off the mites. Put the bedding through a short cycle in the tumble dryer once you take it out to restore its original shape and softness.

- Feathers can cause allergic reactions in the respiratory system. If you have such sensitivities, try an alternative to feather pillows.

## Caring for the Respiratory System with Herbs

There are several ways in which herbs can help to improve and protect respiratory functions and a number of different methods of taking these herbs. The most important types of herbal action and preparation are described below.

### Antiallergic

Herbs can help if you experience allergic respiratory conditions such as asthma and hay fever. Try East Indian walnut (*Albizia lebbeck*) and

Baical skullcap (*Scutellaria baicalensis*). If you suffer from hay fever it is useful to take immune stimulant herbs such as echinacea (*see* chapter 8) regularly, beginning about a week before you expect to start experiencing hay fever symptoms. Continue taking it until the hay fever season is over.

## Antimicrobial

Herbs that help to destroy the microbes that cause sinus, throat and chest infections can have a vital role to play in preventing as well as treating them. If you tend to develop these kinds of infections regularly, perhaps over the winter months, then it is a good idea to take herbal antimicrobials before the problems set in. This can be a useful approach for older people, who are most at risk of developing serious respiratory infections. Important herbs to consider which have a particular affinity for the respiratory system include:

- Elecampane (*Inula hellenium*),
- Garlic (*Allium sativum*),
- Gumplant (*Grindelia camporum*),
- Marsh cudweed (*Gnaphalium uliginosum*),
- Rosemary (*Rosmarinus officinalis*),
- Sage (*Salvia officinalis*),
- Thyme (*Thymus vulgaris*).

## Antioxidants

Antioxidants with particular affinity for the chest include rosemary, sage and thyme (*see* chapter 6).

## Antispasmodic

Respiratory antispasmodics are helpful in improving conditions such as coughs and asthma. They relax the muscles surrounding the respiratory tract and the bronchial tubes. The most broadly useful antispasmodic of this type is thyme.

## Antitussive

Antitussives are herbs that reduce or stop coughing. Although this can be a good approach, it is not always a suitable way of treating coughs. It is useful for dry, irritating, non-productive coughs (meaning where there is no coughing up of mucus), but not for productive coughing (producing mucus) because it is important to allow the sputum to be brought up the mucociliary escalator and removed from the body or burnt up in the stomach. Using antitussives to control an irritable cough for brief periods of time can sometimes be useful. Excellent antitussive herbs include wild cherry (*Prunus serotina*) and coltsfoot (*Tussilago farfara*).

## Demulcent

These are herbs that have the ability to form gel-like preparations when mixed with water. The gel has a soothing effect when it comes into contact with inflamed areas such as sore throats. Some demulcent herbs are also able to soothe the lungs and are very useful for relieving inflamed chests in coughs and infections. Important herbal demulcents include marshmallow leaves (*Althaea officinalis*) and mullein (*Verbascum thapsus*).

## Expectorant

Expectorant herbs are among the most effective and important in promoting good respiratory health. They improve the defensive mechanisms of the system by enhancing the quality of the mucus lining the respiratory tract and by promoting the work of the mucociliary escalator in quickly and efficiently removing pollutants and infective agents from the body. Regular use may help to prevent allergic conditions, infections and possibly even cancers in this area. Effective expectorant herbs include angelica (*Angelica archangelica*), aniseed (*Pimpinella anisum*), fennel (*Foeniculum vulgare*) and thyme (*Thymus vulgare*).

## Lymphatic

Permanently or recurrently enlarged lymph nodes in the neck are always a symptom that you should explore with your doctor or herbal practitioner. Some people experience this problem along with chronic respiratory congestion or allergy. In such cases, herbs that help to stimulate and drain the lymphatic system can be of great benefit. The most useful herbs for this include cleavers (*Galium aparine*), echinacea (*Echinachea purpurea*), marigold (*Calendula officinalis*) and sweet violet (*Viola odorata*).

## Mucous membrane trophorestoratives

Herbs in this group improve the performance of the membranes which produce mucus. They are excellent to take if you suffer from sore or inflammatory conditions, and especially if you have problems with catarrh. The two most useful herbs of this type are ground ivy (*Glechoma hederacea*) and ribwort plantain (*Plantago lanceolata*).

## General herbal support

If you need general support for the respiratory system, a good general-purpose tea to take as a tonic for the airways is as follows:

10g cloves (*Syzygium aromaticum*)
30g fennel seeds (*Foeniculum vulgare*)
15g ground ivy leaves (*Glechoma hederacea*)
10g mullein leaves (*Verbascum thapsus*)
15g spearmint (*Mentha spicata*)
20g thyme leaves (*Thymus vulgare*)

The above mix adds up to 100g; this amount will provide about a week's treatment. The tea should be made by infusion. This is a pleasant tea that will warm the circulation of the lungs, reduce catarrh, improve expectoration and help prevent infection.

To make the infusion pour 250ml (a mug full) of water that has just boiled over 2 teaspoons of the herbs, cover over and leave to brew for 5 minutes, then stir, strain and drink. Take the tea 2–3 times a day. You can brew the infusion in a teapot or in a mug with a saucer over the top to prevent the volatile oils escaping.

## Steam inhalation

Inhaling steam containing tiny droplets of volatile oils from respiratory herbs with antimicrobial, antispasmodic and expectorant properties can be excellent if you have congested sinuses, coughs and colds, or general catarrhal problems. For making the inhalation you can use dried herbs or the volatile oils (also known as essential oils or aromatherapy oils) extracted from the herbs.

The method for an aromatic inhalation using volatile oils is described here. The same method can be used substituting the oils with a small handful of the same herbs in dried form.

Boil a kettle of water and pour into a suitable large container. Leave the water to cool for 2 minutes (using the water immediately can cause the oils to be too strong when inhaled). Then add 5–10 drops of volatile oil, sprinkled on the surface of the water. Now place your head over the bowl at a safe distance and inhale for 5–10 minutes or until you feel you have had enough.

To increase the potency of the inhalation you can place a towel over your head and the bowl, so creating an enclosed steam chamber. If you use the towel method, cover your face with the towel as you move away from the steam and rest for a minute like this before removing the towel completely. This makes for a gentler and more relaxing transition from hot, steamy air to the cooler air in the room.

A good blend for an inhalation for general catarrhal congestion of the chest, nose or sinuses is:

3 drops eucalyptus (*Eucalyptus globulus*)
3 drops thyme (*Thymus vulgaris*)
4 drops peppermint (*Mentha piperita*)

*Caution*

When the lining of the nose and throat is very inflamed, volatile oil inhalations can be irritating to the membranes. If you are an asthmatic you may find that your breathing problems are exacerbated by inhalations and you should use them with care.

## Chest rubs

Chest rubs are used to treat chest infections as well as for improving general respiratory health and preventing respiratory disease as they stimulate circulation to the respiratory muscles and boost immune-system activity and expectoration. It is a good idea to apply regular chest rubs if you have catarrhal problems, and as a preventive treatment during the winter months or at other times when you are at increased risk of developing coughs, colds and chest infections.

A chest rub consists of a carrier oil (such as almond oil) mixed with one or more volatile oils. The ratio of volatile oil to fixed oil can vary but in general it is advisable to use a volatile oil content in the region of 1–2%. This means that if you make up 100ml of chest rub you will use 1 or 2ml of volatile oils with 99 or 98ml of carrier oil. Volatile oils usually come in dropper bottles so it is important to know that 1ml is equivalent to 20 drops. You can make up a chest rub in 100 or 200ml bottles at a time. It is best to keep your rub in glass bottles as these retain the properties of the oils better than plastic; volatile oils can also corrode plastic containers.

Chest rubs should be massaged over the sternum (breastbone) on the front of the chest, and between the shoulder blades on the back. It is not necessary to massage over the whole of the chest. An excellent chest rub for general use is:

20 drops gully gum (*Eucalyptus smithii*)
20 drops thyme (*Thymus vulgaris*)
100ml sweet almond oil

Mix the ingredients and store in a glass bottle, then rub over the chest each morning and evening.

*Caution*

Most people will tolerate most volatile oils if properly diluted with a carrier oil. If you have sensitive skin it is wise to patch test a small area of skin on your arm or leg to see if there is a reaction before massaging over a wider area. Always avoid volatile oils coming into contact with the eyes, mouth and genitals, even when they have been diluted. Remember to wash your hands immediately after applying the chest rub to avoid accidentally touching these areas. Cover bed linen with an old sheet or towels to avoid staining, and let oils fully absorb into the skin before dressing as otherwise they may damage clothes.

# Herbs for the Respiratory System

There are many medicinal plants that can give positive results for respiratory health. Those described below are amongst the most useful.

## Cloves

Cloves (*Syzygium aromaticum*) are the dried flower buds from the clove tree. They have very good antimicrobial and expectorant properties and warm the circulation to the lungs. They are an excellent addition to winter drinks to prevent infections and ward off chills. The best way to take them is to add half a dozen cloves to hot drinks, such as a mix of hot water and lemon juice, or in combination with some of the herbs mentioned below. Clove volatile oil makes an effective decongestant and antibacterial inhalation using 2–3 drops to a bowl of hot water.

## Elecampane

Elecampane (*Inula hellenium*) is a tall European herb with large leaves and bright yellow flowers. Its roots are used in medicine and they contain a strongly antimicrobial and expectorant volatile oil. They also have a bitter taste which stimulates the digestion. Elecampane is a fabulous herb to use to protect the lungs in times of increased risk of developing coughs and colds – if everyone in the office has nasty coughs then elecampagne will help to keep you from joining them. It should be taken as a decoction, using 1–2 teaspoons per cup and, because of its bitterness, it is best combined with a more pleasant-tasting herb such as fennel or liquorice.

## Eucalyptus

There are at least 450 different species of eucalyptus, of which blue gum (*Eucalyptus globulus*) is probably the most commonly used as a medicine. Although the dried leaves can be made into an infusion and used therapeutically, it is the volatile oil that is more widely used. Inhalations and chest rubs made with eucalyptus are very helpful in easing catarrhal congestion, stimulating circulation and boosting immune activity in the respiratory tract. Gully gum (*Eucalyptus smithii*) provides a remarkably gentle type of eucalyptus oil that is particularly useful for chest rubs.

## Fennel

Fennel (*Foeniculum vulgare*) has warming and relaxing effects on the lungs, helping to relieve congestion, thin the mucus and bring up phlegm. Two plants closely related to fennel, angelica (*Angelica archangelica*) and aniseed (*Pimpinella anisum*), have similar properties. All three have antimicrobial properties and are soothing for coughs. Fennel makes a pleasant tea and is an excellent herb to take regularly to improve both respiratory and digestive functions.

Take fennel as a tea using 2 teaspoons to a cup and preparing by infusion. The seeds are the part of the plant that is used and it helps to crush them lightly in a pestle and mortar before using in order to release the volatile oil. Fresh fennel leaves chopped fine and infused can also be used and are very refreshing. Fennel tea is widely available in teabag form.

## Liquorice

As well as being commonly given to complement the activities of adaptogenic herbs, liquorice (*Glycyrrhiza glabra*) has anti-inflammatory, demulcent and expectorant qualities. It is soothing, lubricating and relaxing for the airways, and can be taken during periods of stress and tension if you tend towards developing coughs and colds at such times. Due to its soothing effects, it is useful for singers, teachers and anyone who has to use their voice a great deal. It is wise to avoid taking this herb if you have high blood pressure since liquorice can exacerbate this condition.

Take liquorice by decocting 2 teaspoons of the roots in a mug of water. Drink 1–2 cups a day. Liquorice combines very well with thyme or elecampagne to broaden its effects.

## Mullein

The leaves and flowers of mullein (*Verbascum thapsus*) are wonderfully silky soft to the touch and they impart this quality to teas made from them. Mullein makes a pleasant demulcent herbal tea that can be used to protect the mucous membranes of the airways from harmful pollution and dry atmospheres. Use 1 teaspoon of the flowers or leaves per cup, prepare by infusion, and drink 1–3 cups a day. It is a good herbal tea to carry with you in a thermos if you have to work in dusty or hot and dry environments.

## Ribwort plantain

Ribwort plantain (*Plantago lanceolata*) is an excellent antiallergic and mucous membrane trophorestorative plant. It is useful if you have asthma, or suffer from hay fever, catarrh or sinusitis. The leaves of ribwort plantain contain aucubin, a substance with antibiotic properties. This herb can be of help if you find that you are having recurrent irritating coughs or raised lymph glands. It is also good for chronic middle ear and nasal congestion. Take 2 teaspoons of the leaves per cup and prepare by infusion. Elderflower (*Sambucus nigra*) is a good herb to take in combination with ribwort plantain due to its immune-stimulating action (*see* page 123) and it also has an ability to relieve mucus congestion in the airways.

## Thyme

This Mediterranean herb (*Thymus vulgaris*) has a multitude of uses for the respiratory system. It can help treat many conditions, including sore throats, catarrh, recurrent coughs and colds, bronchitis and asthma, and it has even been used for whooping cough. It is unsurpassed as a protective and enhancing herb for the respiratory system. Thyme improves circulation to the airways, thereby providing the energy and nutrients the lungs need from the blood and facilitating the efficient exchange of respiratory gases. It enhances the removal of wastes from the lungs via the circulation by its expectorant action, thus preventing the build-up of toxic chemicals in the respiratory tract. It is a strong antioxidant and may play a role in helping to prevent lung cancer. Additionally, thyme helps to prevent lung infections, loosens catarrhal congestion and relaxes the alveoli in the lungs, helping to maximise our breathing capacity.

As a general preventive the leaves and flowers of thyme are best taken as a tea, but the dried or fresh herb can also be used as an inhalation, as can the volatile oil. Some more details about this fantastic respiratory herb are provided below.

## KEY HERB FOR THE RESPIRATORY SYSTEM

## THYME

**Scientific name** *Thymus vulgaris*

**Plant family** Lamiaceae (Mint family)

**Type of plant** Small perennial shrub.

**Part used** Leaves, stem and flowers.

**Phytochemicals** Flavonoids; volatile oil (containing carvacrol and thymol).

**Actions** Antioxidant; antimicrobial, antispasmodic, expectorant.

**Indications** Asthma; catarrh; cough (wet, productive coughs); sore throat.

**Preparations** The tea is made by infusion – use 2 teaspoons per cup and drink 1–3 times a day. The dried herb or volatile oil can be used to make an inhalation. Gargling with the tea is useful for sore throats.

**Combinations** Combines well with liquorice, mullein and fennel.

**Cautions** Thyme is a culinary herb and considered to be very safe. It was traditionally used to treat a number of gynaecological conditions and it is probably wise to keep the use of thyme to a minimum in pregnancy.

**Conservation** Thyme is widely cultivated for culinary and medicinal use but overharvesting of wild populations has endangered some thyme species locally in parts of Europe.

# Chapter 12

# HERBS FOR BONES, MUSCLES AND SKIN –

## Supple joints, radiant skin

The bones, muscles and skin – the musculoskeletal system – combine to provide the structure of the body and the mechanical components for movement. The bones provide the framework to which the muscles attach and they are overlaid by the protective coating of the skin. Although the bones, muscles and skin do have largely mechanical roles to play, they are more complex than this, and our health and well-being are greatly enhanced when they function to their full potential.

## The Musculoskeletal System

### Bones

The most obvious role of bones is that they form the skeleton which provides our structure, enabling us to stand upright, and that they provide a cage to protect our vital organs. Bones are also the supports to which muscles attach and the storage areas for minerals and energy (which can be produced from the fat cells in the bone marrow). Additionally, some bones contain cells that can produce red and white blood cells.

#### Problems in the bones and joints

One of the major problems with bones is that they can break. Weakening of the bone due to osteoporosis can mean that bones fracture more easily. This is a condition that concerns many people, especially as they grow older and it is most significant in our joints. There are several types of joint but they are all points of mechanical articulation. Joints can suffer from wear and tear over the years, leading to osteoarthritis, which can be a very painful and disabling condition when it is severe. Osteoarthritis occurs when the layer of cartilage covering the tips of bones becomes eroded.

Rheumatoid arthritis also attacks the joints but it is an autoimmune disease where the body starts to attack its own joints. Other joint problems include gout, ankylosing spondylitis, psoriatic arthritis, juvenile arthritis and a range of others that are named after particular activities or occupations, such as tennis elbow (lateral epicondylitis), golfer's elbow (medial epicondylitis), housemaid's knee (prepatellar bursitis) and student's elbow (olecranon bursitis).

Many people take anti-inflammatories for joint and muscle problems; most commonly these are non-steroidal anti-inflammatory drugs (NSAIDs) such as ibuprofen. NSAIDs were developed to replace aspirin, which can cause bleeding from the stomach.

## Muscles

Our muscles enable us to move by contracting and relaxing, pulling against the bones which work as levers. In movement, muscles also generate heat to keep us warm and they pump blood through the veins to the heart.

Muscles are spread throughout the body and exist in several types. Most familiar are those that are attached to the skeleton, enabling us to move. A different kind of muscle, called smooth muscle, lines the walls of structures inside the body such as the blood vessels and intestines, and this enables movement inside the body. The heart is made from a specialised type of muscle known as cardiac muscle.

### Muscle problems

Several problems involving the joints can also involve the muscles, and these include tennis elbow, frozen shoulder and repetitive strain injury. Lower back pain, which can involve muscles, joints or both, is an increasingly common problem. We tend to use the words *arthritis* and *rheumatism* to refer to joint problems; the term *muscular rheumatism* was formerly used to describe muscle pains that did not involve bone problems. Beyond bone fractures, osteoarthritis and particular problems affecting the bones or muscles specifically (such as Paget's disease of the bones), bone and muscular problems tend to occur in association with each other. For example, rheumatoid arthritis involves inflammation of both the joints and the muscles.

Fibromyalgia, a condition of widespread muscular tenderness, and muscular weakness and fatigue associated with chronic fatigue syndrome (ME) are both problems commonly encountered. Another large area of muscular problems can be grouped under the heading 'sports injuries'.

Muscles and skin are both sensitive to psychological influences. Tension and stress can lead to stiffness in the muscles, causing pain and headaches. The muscles contract and relax in response to nerve action, and our nervous system is clearly in tune with our mental or emotional state.

## Skin

The term 'skin', in this context, also includes hair and nails, since these are part of our outer covering. Our skin has a hard, waxy outer layer (the epidermis) which protects the body from abrasion, infection, dehydration and ultraviolet radiation from the sun. The skin also:

- Regulates body temperature by sweating;
- Picks up sensations of temperature, touch, pressure and pain;
- Produces vitamin D (upon exposure of the skin to sunlight);
- Provides part of the immune system;
- Forms a channel for detoxification.

## Skin problems

A wide range of conditions can affect the skin, including acne, cellulite, eczema, psoriasis, and skin cancer.

The skin can reveal our emotions through blushing and, in conjunction with changes in the muscles, by our facial expressions. The accumulated effects of age, environment, diet and lifestyle can be read in our faces. Because our face is our most noticeable feature, skin conditions involving the face can severely affect our self-confidence – a skin condition such as acne can badly affect ones self-image.

Although sunlight is necessary on our skin to synthesise vitamin D, too much ultraviolet (UV) radiation can burn the skin and play a part in the development of skin cancer. In hot, bright weather one should avoid prolonged exposure to the sun.

# Caring for Your Bones, Muscles and Skin

In order to maintain healthy, pain-free joints and relaxed muscles, and to promote the integrity and vibrancy of the skin, it is necessary to pay careful attention to your diet, exercise and relaxation.

## Diet

We all need a diet containing a healthy balance of nutrients to nourish our bones, muscles and skin. Deficiencies of specific nutrients can cause chronic problems, contributing to conditions such as dry skin, dandruff and the effects of ageing on the skin. In addition, there are some foods that can make particular conditions worse and so they should be eaten only in small amounts or avoided completely. In order to function at their best the bones, muscles and skin need a good supply of vitamins, minerals, essential fatty acids and protein. (*See* pages 191–2 for a list of foods and herbs that supply these nutrients.)

Protein is vital for forming and maintaining bone, muscle and skin, and we should eat high-quality protein that provides a broad spectrum of amino acids. Good sources of protein include soya products, fish, whole grains and pulses such as chick peas and red kidney beans. It you are a vegetarian who does not eat fish it is important to combine proteins from both pulses and grains to ensure that you get the full range of amino acids, consuming them within 24 hours of each other. Nutrients that work alongside proteins and improve their uptake and performance in the body include chromium, folic acid and manganese. Vitamins B1 (thiamine) and B6 (pyridoxine) are essential to help the body form collagen, the main connective tissue protein in the body. In addition to this, advice is given below for specific conditions.

**Osteoporosis** – Bones are made up mainly of collagen fibres and bone salts. The bone salts are minerals and trace minerals including boron, calcium, magnesium and potassium. Thinning of the bones in osteoporosis is of concern to all, but particularly to women after the menopause, when the protective effects of oestrogen on bone density are decreased. The key to tackling osteoporosis is prevention. The risk of developing this condition can be decreased by taking regular aerobic exercise and having a diet rich in the nutrients necessary for achieving good bone density, especially boron, calcium, copper, magnesium, manganese, and vitamins A and D.

**Rheumatoid arthritis and osteoarthritis** – Gamma-linolenic acid (GLA) and omega-3 essential fatty acids can be of benefit in relieving the symptoms of rheumatoid arthritis and osteoarthritis. GLA provides the starting material for the production of anti-inflammatory prostaglandins and so can help reduce pain and discomfort. Fish oils are of particular use in reducing inflammation in rheumatoid arthritis. Additional support in improving rheumatoid arthritis can be found by taking vitamin E (for its antioxidant properties) and a multimineral supplement including copper, selenium and zinc.

**Skin care** – Skin cells are continuously being replaced and this means that the skin can quickly reflect ill health and nutritional deficiencies. As well as a good general protein intake, skin nutrition is founded on optimal intakes of water, fruit and vegetables (antioxidants), omega-3 essential fatty acids, vitamins A, C, B6 and B12, folic acid and zinc.

**Angular stomatitis** – A common skin problem experienced is cracking of the corners of the mouth (angular stomatitis) and this reflects a deficiency in vitamin B2 and iron. To counter this condition, take supplements of these nutrients and ensure that you get plenty of rest – it is likely that you have become run down. If the condition persists you should see a herbal practitioner or doctor.

**Dry skin** – If you have constantly dry skin this can be helped by taking a GLA supplement (such as evening primrose oil), decreasing your intake of saturated fat (for instance from meat, eggs and dairy products), while increasing polyunsaturated fat intake (found in vegetables, nuts, seeds, seed oils like sesame, sunflower and safflower, and oily fish), and ensuring you regularly consume food sources of vitamins A, C and E, and zinc. Dry nails and hair can benefit from consuming foods that are high in biotin.

**Dandruff** – Dandruff can be improved by eating foods containing vitamin A and consuming omega-3 essential fatty acids. In all dry skin disorders it is essential to remember to drink enough water – 1.5–2 litres per day depending on your age, weight and the environmental temperature.

**Acne, eczema and psoriasis** – Gamma-linolenic acid and omega-3 essential fatty acids can have significant benefits if you have acne, eczema or psoriasis. In each of these conditions it is important to ensure you are getting adequate amounts of foods containing vitamins A, C and E, and selenium and zinc. Acne is also aided by eating soluble fibre rich foods, raw fruit and vegetables, and oily fish. Omega-3 essential fatty acids can also help with problems with hair loss and poor wound healing.

**Ageing skin** – With ageing and exposure to the elements (particularly the wind and sun), the skin can become less elastic and more dry and wrinkled. To reduce these effects follow a diet rich in antioxidants (which prevent damage to skin cells), polyunsaturated fats, good-quality protein, vitamins A, B6, C and E, and the trace minerals selenium and zinc. It is also important to drink sufficient quantities of water.

The following table shows food sources for the essential nutrients mentioned above.

| Nutrient | Good Sources |
| --- | --- |
| Biotin | Soya, whole wheat, oats, mushrooms, avocado. |
| Boron | Cabbage, dates, almonds, pulses, apples, raisins. |
| Calcium | Soya products (e.g. tofu), cabbage, kale, yoghurt, fennel (as a vegetable), broccoli, salmon, oranges, almonds. |
| Chromium | Lentils, wholewheat bread, chicken, potatoes, green peppers, apples. |
| Copper | Lentils, chick peas, kidney beans, sunflower seeds, walnuts, almonds, dried apricots. |
| Fish oils (which are rich in the omega-3 essential fatty acids EPA and DPA) | Halibut, herring, mackerel, salmon, sardines, tuna. |
| Folic acid (also known as *folate*) | Kidney beans, mung beans, dark leafy green vegetables (e.g. cabbage, broccoli, kale), soya products, lentils, walnuts. |
| Gamma linolenic-acid (GLA) | Evening primrose, borage and blackcurrant oils. |
| Magnesium | Brown rice, sunflower seeds, wholewheat bread, lentils, walnuts, almonds. |

| Nutrient | Good Sources |
| --- | --- |
| Manganese | Pecan nuts, Brazil nuts, buckwheat, oatmeal, hazelnuts, dried fruit (e.g. apricots, figs), walnuts, brown rice. |
| Omega-3 essential fatty acids | Flax (linseed) and hemp oils. Fish oils. |
| Potassium | Butter beans, haricot beans, lentils, bananas, spinach, wholewheat bread, fresh vegetables, potatoes. |
| Selenium | Tuna, herrings, Brazil nuts, sardines, oats, barley, garlic, brown rice. |
| Vitamin A (from beta-carotene) | Green leafy vegetables (such as cabbage, spinach, kale, broccoli), carrots, sweet potatoes, pumpkins, apricots, peaches. |
| Vitamin B1 (thiamine) | Sunflower seeds, pine nuts, Brazil nuts, pinto beans, split peas, millet. |
| Vitamin B2 (riboflavin) | Almonds, mushrooms, millet, chilli peppers, spinach, yoghurt. |
| Vitamin B6 (pyridoxine) | Sunflower seeds, walnuts, lentils, lima beans, brown rice, hazelnuts. |
| Vitamin B12 (cobalamin) | Organ meats, sardines, salmon, tuna, lamb. |
| Vitamin C | Red chilli peppers, guavas, kale, parsley, broccoli, Brussels sprouts, watercress, oranges, lemon juice, grapefruit, elderberries. |
| Vitamin D | This vitamin is produced by the action of sunlight on the skin. It is also in mackerel, salmon, herring and dark-green leafy vegetables. |
| Vitamin E | Polyunsaturated vegetable oils, seeds, nuts, whole grains, avocados, green leafy vegetables. |
| Zinc | Pumpkin seeds, ginger root, pecan nuts, split peas, Brazil nuts, oats, lima beans, almonds, walnuts. |

## Foods to avoid

In **osteoarthritis** there is often a food sensitivity to plants in the nightshade family (Solanaceae), such as potatoes, tomatoes, aubergines and peppers; this may be a side effect from taking NSAIDs for pain relief since these may damage the gut, allowing food allergens to get into the bloodstream.

In **rheumatoid arthritis** it is important to avoid foods that can exacerbate inflammation, such as red meat and cheese, and to steer clear of foods that are high in waste products, such as organ meats and shellfish, since the wastes can accumulate around inflamed joints and provoke further inflammation.

In **gout**, avoid foods containing purines (since these chemicals break down to produce uric acid, which is the chemical responsible for causing gout); these are present in red meat, organ meats, shellfish, herring, sardines, mackerel, anchovies and lentils.

In cases of **muscular tightness** (perhaps triggered by stress) or weakness and fatigue (as in chronic fatigue syndrome) it is wise to avoid drinks containing caffeine, such as coffee and cola, since these can increase muscle contractions and impair muscular energy production.

To improve **skin tone**, it is wise to avoid highly processed foods, foods high in sugar, salt, artificial flavourings, colourings and saturated fats. In **acne** it is particularly important to avoid saturated fat consumption (including chocolate and hydrogenated margarine), sugary foods and salty foods (such as salted peanuts), and to keep away from foods containing hormones such as dairy milk.

In **psoriasis** around 16% of sufferers have an allergy to gluten. Removing gluten-rich grains (wheat, rye, barley) from the diet can clear all symptoms. (To find out whether you might have this allergy contact your doctor for an anti-gliadin antibody test).

A number of foods are known to exacerbate **eczema** and should be avoided if you tend to this condition; they include dairy milk, eggs, cheese, chocolate, oranges and orange juice, fizzy drinks, nuts and food additives.

## Exercise

It is important to build up bone density with aerobic exercise (such as running, cycling and swimming). Aerobic exercise is also crucial in achieving and maintaining an ideal weight. This is important for relieving pressure on the joints, especially the hips and knees, which in turn reduces the risk of developing osteoarthritis.

Regular exercise improves muscular strength, endurance and flexibility. It also improves energy reserves and helps the removal of waste products from the muscles. Exercise stimulates circulation to the skin and this stimulates its nutrition and detoxification.

## Relaxation

Relaxation is important for the:

- Skeletal muscle – reducing back pain and headaches;
- Cardiac muscle, especially if prone to palpitations and angina;
- Smooth muscle – lowering high blood pressure and calming irritable bowel syndrome.

Physical, emotional and mental stress causes muscle stiffness and tenderness, making massage an effective treatment. It is a great idea to receive massage regularly (say, once a week) from a practitioner, friend or partner. Short courses in basic massage techniques are widely available.

Although rest is not necessarily an equivalent to relaxation, sufficient good-quality sleep is important to the whole body. If we are not rested, it is unlikely we can relax.

Stress also affects the skin – psoriasis particularly can flare up due to stressful situations – so relaxation will be helpful.

# Herbal Actions for the Bones, Muscles and Skin

Several categories of herbs offer possibilities in helping us to care for the bones, muscles and skin in addition to the advice given above.

## Anti-inflammatory

Anti-inflammatory herbs such as devil's claw (*Harpagophytum procumbens*), salai guggal (*Boswellia serrata*) and the spice turmeric (*Curcuma longa*) can relieve muscular and joint pain and discomfort and may be particularly useful if you suffer from occasional sore joints or muscles, helping to prevent further progression of the condition.

## Stimulants and relaxants

Circulatory stimulants and relaxants can bring positive results when used to help muscular disorders. Circulatory stimulants, such as rosemary (*Rosmarinus officinalis*), improve muscular nutrition and detoxification. Muscular relaxants such as cramp bark (*Viburnum opulus*) and kava (*Piper methysticum*) can combat the debilitating effects of stress and tension, helping the muscles to cope with the strain put upon the body.

## Depuratives

Depuratives are herbs that improve skin conditions by enhancing detoxification processes. These plants were once known as 'blood cleansers'. Depurative herbs are helpful to take if you regularly experience skin problems such as boils and regular pustular spots, as well as acne, eczema or psoriasis. Such herbs include cleavers (*Galium aparine*), Oregon grape root (*Mahonia aquifolium*) and birch leaves (*Betula* species). Detoxifying and cleansing herbs are also helpful for joint inflammations such as rheumatoid arthritis; examples include a mixture of celery seeds (*Apium graveolens*) and dandelion leaves (*Taraxacum officinale*).

## Nervines

These are herbs that calm, nourish and strengthen the nervous system, and skullcap (*Scutellaria lateriflora*) is one of the most helpful herbs for dealing with nervous system involvement with skin conditions; valerian (*Valeriana officinalis*) is one of the best herbs for working on this level to treat tense muscles. (For more on nervines, *see* chapter 14.)

# Herbs for the Bones, Muscles and Skin

The herbs given below are among the most beneficial for supporting the functions of the bones, muscles and skin, and for boosting their performance.

## Cleavers

Cleavers (*Galium aparine*) is a European weed, also known as goosegrass and sticky Willie. It has little hairs that can make it easy to hook on to clothing, hence the references to 'cleaving' and being sticky. Although little researched, this plant is widely used in British herbal medicine, valued for its gentleness, safety and effectiveness. It is considered to improve the drainage of the lymphatic system, relieving congestion in the lymph nodes. Cleavers has a cooling and moisturising effect on hot, dry skin problems. A tea made from this herb may prove very useful if you have eczema, seborrhoeic dermatitis or a tendency towards dry, hot or red skin problems. If you develop irritable red skin in reaction to heat (such as hot baths or hot weather), or so-called 'prickly heat', this herb can be very soothing.

To make cleavers tea, use 2 teaspoons of the dried herb (leaf and stems) per cup, make by infusion, and take 2–3 cups each day as required. The fresh herb can be used at a dosage of a small handful of the herb per cup, again made by infusion. Fresh young cleavers can also be added to soups as a spring cleansing herb.

# Devil's claw

Devil's claw (*Harpagophytum procumbens*) is well known for treating inflammatory joint problems such as osteoarthritis. It is a South African plant also commonly known as 'grapple plant'. The main active constituent is a glycoside called harpagoside which has anti-inflammatory properties. The plant has a bitter taste and this indictaes that it has a potential extra role in improving digestive functions, but it should be avoided by anybody who has a duodenal or stomach ulcer. Devil's claw offers an alternative painkiller for people who are dependent on non-steroidal anti-inflammatory drugs (NSAIDs) such as ibuprofen. Devil's claw does not cause the side effects associated with NSAIDs and is therefore a healthier product to use. Before switching from NSAIDs, you should talk to a doctor and herbal practitioner to make sure this is the right thing for your own circumstances.

Devil's claw can be taken as a decoction of the roots at a dosage of 2 teaspoons of the root per cup taken 3 times a day between meals, or as an enteric-coated capsule at a dose equivalent to a total of 3–6g of the dried root per day.

Since devil's claw is considered an endangered species, you should try to use supplies of this herb that come from certified sustainable sources.

# Evening primrose oil and hemp oil

Evening primrose oil (*Oenethera biennis*) is an excellent source of gamma-linolenic acid, which has good anti-inflammatory activity and can improve vascular and nerve function in diabetics. It also has anti-allergic properties. The combination of these qualities means that evening primrose oil (EPO) has good relieving and preventive actions for joint conditions such as rheumatoid arthritis and skin conditions such as eczema. EPO can be taken in capsules at a dose of around 2.5–5g per day (equivalent to 250–500mg GLA per day) for general enhancing and preventive activity. EPO is considered to be safe and well tolerated, although there has been some concern that it should be avoided by epileptics. Until conclusive research has been carried out it would be wise to avoid this oil at the present time if you do suffer from any form of epilepsy.

Hemp oil (*Cannabis sativa*) is my favourite source of omega-3 essential fatty acids because it is well tolerated and very effective. One teaspoon a day of hemp oil can be taken as part of a healthy dietary regime to improve skin tone, reduce skin allergies, and prevent and treat arthritis. This type of essential fatty acids also has protective effects for the heart and circulation. It is important to take your hemp oil unheated, for example in salad dressing or spread on bread in place of butter or margarine; some people are happy to take it neat from a teaspoon, but not everybody enjoys the taste. Hemp oil is cold pressed from hemp seeds and has none of the intoxicating effects caused by consumption of the cannibinoids in hemp leaves.

## Kava

Kava (*Piper methysticum*) is a native of the islands that make up the region of Oceania, such as New Guinea and Fiji, and is a member of the pepper family (culinary black pepper – *Piper nigrum*). Indigenous use of this plant is both as a medicine and as a sacred herb in social and religious ceremonies. When prepared as a ceremonial drink it engenders a sense of well-being and euphoria. Part of this effect is retained in medicinal preparations, which engender feelings of calm, contentment and reduced anxiety. Kava is also an excellent muscle relaxant and is ideal for easing tension and stiffness in muscles due to stress and conditions such as tension headaches.

Some concerns have been expressed about a small number of reported cases of adverse effects. These have been linked to the use of industrial preparations that were high in kavalactones (the main active chemical constituents in kava) and that differ greatly from traditional preparations which are considered to be safe – long-term use of kava in Oceania over thousands of years is not associated with any significant medical problems. At the time of writing, however, kava has been banned by the UK government, and its use is not currently permitted under UK law.

## Marigold

As well as possessing an immune enhancing capacity (*see* chapter 8), Marigold (*Calendula officinalis*) is an important herb for the skin and muscles. It is a good anti-inflammatory herb for both these tissues and aids the reduction in joint inflammation. It also stimulates the lymphatic system and helps with boils and pustular spots on the skin. Externally, creams made with the flowers are soothing and healing to the skin and have antibacterial and antifungal properties useful with conditions such as athlete's foot and ringworm. Marigold cream is also good for sprains, bites and bruises, making it an excellent general first-aid cream.

Calendula (marigold) flower tea may be right for you if you are prone to recurrent skin infections, stiff joints or sore, tight muscles. The tea is made by using 1 heaped teaspoon of the flower petals to a cup of water and preparing this by infusion. Take 1–3 cups a day as needed. Commercial marigold creams are widely available.

# Nettle

Nettle leaves (*Urtica dioica*) provide a very good tonic herb for the joints, muscles and skin. They have detoxifying and anti-inflammatory effects that are particularly useful for relieving the symptoms of osteoarthritis and several skin problems including boils and acne. Beyond this, nettles are considered a general preventive cleansing agent for the bones, muscles and skin, helping to remove toxic wastes from these tissues and acting to protect them from future disease.

I would urge caution if you have eczema. In some cases, eczema responds well to nettles, but in others it can be exacerbated by them. Nettle is a nutrient herb containing vitamins C, B and K and minerals. It also contains silicon, which is important for bone development.

Nettle leaves can be taken as a tea, using 1–2 teaspoons to a cup prepared by infusion and taking 1–3 cups per day. The fresh young leaves can also be taken in soups like cleavers. Cut off the top 2 or 3 pairs of leaves and add to spring soups. They combine very well with seaweed and, be reassured, the sting is neutralised once the leaves have been cooked.

# Oregon grape

Oregon grape (*Mahonia aquifolium*) is a North American shrub that is grown widely in Europe as an ornamental plant. It has yellow flowers and roots which contain active chemicals called berberine alkaloids. The roots are used medicinally and have anti-inflammatory, detoxifying and immune stimulating attributes. This plant has established value in improving skin conditions such as psoriasis and acne, and in calming inflamed joints. It is also a useful herb to include in detoxification mixtures (*see* chapter 5).

Oregon grape tea is prepared by decocting 1 teaspoon of the plant's roots and taking 1–3 cups a day as needed. It combines very well with cleavers.

## Turmeric

Turmeric (*Curcuma longa*) is well known as a spice used in curries, soups, stews and other dishes. It is a vivid deep yellow in colour and needs to be handled with care as it will stain your clothes. Turmeric is an excellent anti-inflammatory, antioxidant and cholesterol-lowering herb. As a medicine, it can be a taken as a powder or a tincture as an effective anti-inflammatory for joint disease, and it can help protect the joints from damage and deterioration.

Try and use turmeric regularly in your cooking to reap benefits from it, but be aware that high doses can have a laxative effect. If you suffer from irritable bowel syndrome or loose bowels, this may not be the most appropriate herb for you, other than in very small amounts.

### KEY HERB FOR THE BONES, MUSCLES AND SKIN

## MARIGOLD

**Scientific name** *Calendula officinalis*

**Plant family** Asteraceae (Daisy family)

**Type of plant** Annual herb.

**Part used** Flowers.

**Phytochemicals** Carotenes; flavonoids; resin.

**Actions** Antibacterial, antifungal, anti-inflammatory, antispasmodic, immune stimulant, lymphatic, vulnerary.

**Indications** Marigold can be taken internally for inflammation of joints, skin disorders such as acne, enlarged lymph nodes, sore or bruised muscles, and inflamed and spastic muscles causing lower back pain. It can be used externally for abscesses, athlete's foot, boils, bruises, dry skin and lips, stings, and to protect the skin against pollution and wounds.

**Preparations** *Tea*: 1 teaspoon of the flower petals to a cup of water and prepared by infusion. Take 1–3 cups a day. *Tincture*: (1:2, 25% alcohol), take 5–10ml per day in water. *External use*: marigold cream (often sold as calendula cream), baths or poultices.

**Combinations** For muscular tension combines well with lavender flowers. For enlarged lymph nodes combines well with cleavers. Externally it combines well with St John's wort oil (*Hypericum perforatum*).

**Cautions** Internal use may sometimes exacerbate eczema. Otherwise, marigold can be considered a very gentle and well-tolerated herb.

**Conservation** Marigold is widely cultivated for medicinal use and you can easily grow your own supplies.

# Chapter 13

# HERBS FOR THE REPRODUCTIVE SYSTEM –

## Improving sexual health and vitality

Changing perspectives on sexuality over time have led to an increase in sexual activity outside marriage, more openness in discussing sexual matters and, more recently, signs of an improved status for same sex relationships within society. At the same time there has been a decrease in the amount of women who breast-feed their children and a reduction in the size of families. Many people are waiting until they are older before starting a family and there are also more options available for fertility treatment. Sexually transmitted infections are still with us although the type of the diseases has changed to some extent.

Over this time, the use of herbal medicines to improve sexual interest and performance has remained undiminished. While there are several herbs that can improve libido and sexual performance, there is much more to the use of herbs in the area of the health of the reproductive system than just this.

Good sexual health depends on much the same factors as optimum health in other areas of the body, including having enough sleep, balancing relaxation and exercise, following a good diet, maintaining an optimum weight, reducing stress, avoiding exposure to pollutants, and enjoying satisfying experiences and relationships.

*Caution*
Although herbs have a tremendous amount to offer in helping to achieve enhanced levels of sexual health, it is important to

be cautious about taking herbs during pregnancy, while breast-feeding or if you are undergoing a conventional fertility treatment, such as IVF. In all these cases you should ensure you consult a doctor and herbal practitioner before taking herbal medicines.

# Key Elements of Sexual Health

## Oestrogen

In women, oestrogen is responsible, most significantly during puberty, for developing the female body shape, including the growth of the breasts, and for the growth of the uterus. It also influences female skin tone and bone strength, as well as helping to regulate the menstrual cycle, together with progesterone, throughout the reproductive years.

In men, oestrogen is produced in small amounts and it can also be created as an intermediate stage in the breakdown of testosterone; it appears to play a role in the development of sperm.

### Decreased oestrogen production

The changes experienced during the menopause and the increased risks of developing osteoporosis after the menopause are both associated with a decrease in oestrogen production. Hormone replacement therapy (HRT) with oestrogen is now routinely offered to many women to treat what is conventionally viewed as a state of oestrogen deficiency.

### Increased oestrogen exposure

Although conventional medicine has placed emphasis on potential problems caused by decreased oestrogen levels; in fact, nowadays both women and men are exposed to higher levels of oestrogen than ever before.

This increase can derive from sources both inside and outside of the body. For women, increased longevity, coupled with having fewer children and breast-feeding less often, means that they are likely to experience ten times as many periods as was once the case. This increase is linked with a raised exposure to oestrogen during the menstrual cycle. Oestrogen is created in the body from fats and so the rise in levels of obesity has also been associated with increased oestrogen exposure. In addition, a diet rich in saturated (mainly animal) fats is linked with increased oestrogen production. Oestrogen is also taken internally through the contraceptive pill and in HRT treatment.

Externally, there are a number of compounds which bear some similarity to oestrogen and can stimulate oestrogen receptors in the body. These include agricultural pesticides and hormones, and soft plastics used in food packaging.

Conditions believed to be caused, at least in part, by excessive oestrogen exposure include:

- Heavy periods,
- Premenstrual syndrome (PMS),
- Longer periods,
- Endometriosis,
- Fibroids,
- Fibrocystic breast disease,
- Breast and endometrial cancer,
- Prostate cancer,
- Male infertility.

Reducing oestrogen exposure can be a very important activity for all of us in helping to prevent such conditions. Reduction can be achieved by:

- Reducing saturated fat intake;
- Eating soluble fibre sources (such as fruit and vegetable skins) to reduce absorption of saturated fats, ensuring that all fruit and vegetables are organically grown where possible;

- Controlling the diet and increasing exercise in order to achieve and maintain an optimum body weight;

- Reducing red meat consumption in favour of fish and poultry, ensuring that all flesh eaten is organically reared whenever possible;

- Keeping milk and dairy consumption to a minimum (*see* page 191 for alternative sources of calcium);

- Consuming plants from the cabbage family (such as broccoli, Brussels sprouts and all types of cabbage) as these enhance the breakdown of oestrogen in the body;

- Avoiding the use of foods wrapped in plastics.

One of the major roles that plants can play in the regulation of oestrogen exposure is by using phytoestrogens.

## Phytoestrogens

Plants do not contain oestrogen, but there are plant compounds, the phytoestrogens, which are capable of exerting a degree of oestrogen-like activity. Such compounds include the isoflavonoids, lignans and saponins. The key point is that phytoestrogens have only mild stimulant actions.

Phytoestrogens are between 160 and 1,000 times weaker than the oestrogen that the body produces. They are technically considered to be 'partial agonists', meaning that they can either stimulate or decrease oestrogen levels in the body depending on the state of oestrogen in an individual. In someone who is in a state of oestrogen excess, the weak phytoestrogens will occupy oestrogen receptor sites, blocking them from being more strongly stimulated by oestrogen itself or by potent oestrogen-like substances. This results in a general decrease in the effects of oestrogen on the body. Conversely, in a low-oestrogen state there is a lack of stimulation of oestrogen receptors. In this case, phyto-estrogens can occupy empty oestrogen receptor sites and, although they produce very weak oestrogen stimulation, this will accumulate sufficiently to cause a significant increase in oestrogenic effects.

In the light of this, it is clear that phytoestrogens will tend to decrease the influence of oestrogen in premenopausal women and increase it in postmenopausal women (when oestrogen levels naturally drop). Because the effects of phytoestrogens are very mild, in either case they will tend to modulate normal oestrogen functioning rather than unduly suppressing or over-stimulating. Through these actions, phytoestrogens may help to prevent conditions of both oestrogen excess and deficiency.

Phytoestrogens are present in a number of grains, seeds, legumes, vegetables and medicinal plants. Some examples of good food sources are:

- Grains (such as oats, barley, rye, rice, buckwheat and millet);
- Seeds (such as alfalfa, pumpkin, sunflower and sesame). The phytoestrogenic properties of many seeds are increased when they are sprouted, especially alfalfa seeds;
- Legumes (such as green peas, chick peas, green beans, kidney beans, split peas, mung beans and soya beans);
- Vegetables (such as Brussels sprouts, potatoes eaten with their skins, carrots, asparagus, beetroot and cabbage).

Medicinal plants containing phytoestrogens include:

- Red clover (*Trifolium pratense*),
- Linseeds (*Linum usitatissimum*),
- Black cohosh (*Cimicifuga racemosa*),
- Korean ginseng (*Panax ginseng*),
- Liquorice (*Glycyrrhiza glabra*),
- Fenugreek (*Trigonella foenum-graecum*).

To harness the benefits of phytoestrogens you should seek to incorporate such foods regularly in your diet. It is wise to ensure that the diet contains adequate levels of food phytoestrogens for general protective effects for the reproductive system and to consult a herbalist before taking medicinal plant phytoestrogens to treat a reproductive-system condition that has become well established.

## Soya

Soya products have been discussed more than any other in relation to plant phytoestrogens. This is because some studies have shown decreased levels of oestrogen-related conditions, such as osteoporosis and prostate and breast cancer, in Asian populations that consume significant quantities of soya products. However, concerns have been raised regarding potential harmful effects of soya, particularly in connection with thyroid disease (which is linked to an iodine deficiency). A diet containing both soya products and seaweed (which is rich in iodince) is very unlikely to result in any thyroid problems.

## The contraceptive pill

The problem with contraception from a natural therapist's point of view is that from a biological perspective it is inherently against nature. Nature wants women to conceive and thus to continue the human species. This is not to say that one should abandon all contraception, just acknowledge that such a powerful natural mechanism as conceiving a child cannot easily be overcome.

There is evidence that several indigenous peoples, including some Native North and South American tribes, have managed to use medicinal plants to temporarily prevent conception, but there is currently no known herb that is proven to be able to perform this function safely and effectively. However, research is being carried out into several herbs that might offer prospects for the future, including a male oral contraceptive pill derived from the neem tree (*Azadirachta indica*).

The oral contraceptive pill for women has had a major impact on modern life, providing us with an effective and reliable means of controlling conception. Like all drugs, though, the pill is not without its potential problems and these include the ability to cause headaches, weight gain and fluid retention. Most seriously, the pill can be involved with causing deep vein thrombosis (DVT) in women smokers who are overweight. There is a very small risk from the pill of having a stroke or heart attack, and of developing breast cancer (the latter only seems to be of relevance in women under 35 who have been long-term pill users). On the positive side, there is some evidence that the contraceptive pill may help prevent cancer of the ovaries and uterus, as well as a number of other conditions.

If you feel that the contraceptive pill is best for you then it will help to supplement the diet with vitamins B2, B6, B12 and C, as well as folic acid, magnesium and zinc, since the levels of these nutrients in the body are commonly lowered by the actions of the pill. Taking B6 can help prevent depression, which some women experience when on the pill and taking vitamin E can help reduce the risk of developing DVT.

The combined oral contraceptive pill (containing both oestrogen and progesterone) can interfere with fat and sugar metabolism and it is associated with increased cholesterol levels and difficulties regulating blood sugar. To counter these effects it is wise to ensure that you have a low saturated and hydrogenated fat diet, and one that is low in high glycaemic index foods (sugar rich and refined carbohydrate foods).

Many women decide to come off the pill, either because they wish to conceive or because they would like to stop taking a hormonal drug. The herb chasteberry (*Vitex agnus-castus*) has proven very useful in helping the body adjust to being without the pill, especially after long-term use.

There has been concern about whether it is advisable to take St John's wort (*Hypericum perforatum*) while also on the pill, following reports of several cases of 'breakthrough bleeding' (unexpected bleeding). Although there have been no actual cases of pregnancy documented, it would be wise not to combine these two medicines until further research has been carried out. If you rely on St John's wort but also take the pill, your options are either to keep the herb

and choose an alternative form of contraception or stay on the pill
and consult a herbal practitioner to find an alternative herb.

## Painful periods

Painful periods (dysmenorrhoea) are one of the most common problems
affecting female reproductive health. For some women the pain may be
so severe that they have to take time off work or school. There are a
number of steps you can take to reduce period pain, including:

- Increasing exercise levels; this helps improve uterine tone
  and circulation and relieve menstrual congestion;
- Avoiding animal fats (meat, eggs and dairy produce); these
  contain arachidonic acid which the body metabolises to
  form inflammatory prostaglandins, which exacerbate period
  pain;
- Consuming essential fatty acids (from evening primrose oil
  and oily fish); these help the body produce alternative
  prostaglandins that have anti-inflammatory effects;
- Taking a calcium and magnesium supplement continuously
  or through the second half of your cycle and through the
  period itself; this will have antispasmodic effects, easing the
  uterine and abdominal muscles;
- Applying a hot water bottle to the lower abdomen; this can
  provide some degree of muscle relaxation during the period
  itself.

Several herbs can help provide relief during painful periods and taken
regularly throughout the cycle may help to prevent pain from
occurring at all:

- Raspberry leaf, chamomile and ginger can all be taken as
  teas;
- Dong quai (*Angelica sinensis*) can be very useful if you
  experience a long menstrual cycle with a weak flow during
  the period itself. It should be avoided if you tend to have
  heavy periods;

- A mixture of black haw (*Viburnum prunifolium*) and wild yam (*Dioscorea villosa*) is often helpful, especially to relieve tight, spastic muscular pain;
- Chasteberry (*Vitex agnus-castus*) can be of major benefit if the period pain follows on from symptoms of premenstrual syndrome (*see* below), but it should be avoided if period pain occurs with no premenstrual syndrome (uncomplicated dysmenorrhoea).

## Premenstrual syndrome (PMS)

Painful periods can occur in conjunction with, or separate from, premenstrual syndrome (PMS). There are several different types of PMS, and their classification is based on the predominant symptom experienced:

- PMS-A – the A stands for anxiety and includes mood changes, such as irritability and rapid changes in mood ('mood swings');
- PMS-C – where there are food cravings; there may also be headaches and dizziness;
- PMS-D – where depression is the key feature; women with this form of PMS may also be tearful and confused;
- PMS-H – hyperhydration, or fluid retention, causing the sensation of bloating and breast tenderness;
- PMS-P – pain, such as cramping abdominal pain, joint pains and back pain.

In many cases, women experience more than one of these categories of symptom. The causes of PMS are not well understood, but there are several things that you can do to help relieve and prevent this condition. Bear in mind that you can combine advice for several types if you experience more than one category of PMS symptom.

## PMS-A

- Follow the advice for reducing oestrogen exposure (*see* pages 205–6) and include phytoestrogens in the diet.
- Take vitamin B complex containing 50mg of vitamin B6 from a few days before the time you would normally expect to start experiencing PMS and continue until the symptoms stop.
- Take a magnesium supplement of 200–800mg per day.
- Take chasteberry drops, 5–20 drops of the 1:1 tincture each morning (*see* page 227 for profile of this herb).
- Select one or two nervine herbs (*see* chapter 14) to treat your own picture of mood disturbance.

## PMS-C

Cravings reflect states of low blood sugar and often manifest as a desire for sugary and refined carbohydrate products, such as chocolates, cakes and, sometimes, alcohol. Cravings may be an attempt by the body to improve mood by eating foods that will stimulate the production of serotonin (a mood-enhancing neurochemical). Indulging these cravings can contribute to water retention and bloating (PMS-H).

- Try to eat foods that contain the amino acid tryptophan (which is used by the body to produce serotonin) as an alternative to sweet foods; tryptophan is contained in such foods as cashew nuts, sunflower seeds, tuna fish and oatmeal.
- Avoid caffeine and salt, keep alcohol intake low and eat foods rich in magnesium, such as nuts, seeds, whole grains and vegetables.
- PMS-C may be associated with Syndrome X (insulin resistance syndrome). For advice on how to address this problem, *see* pages 253–7.

**PMS-H**

- Follow all the advice given for PMS-A.
- Take evening primrose oil and essential fatty acids in the form of fish oils.
- Supplement the diet with vitamin E (400–800 IU per day) if breast tenderness is present.
- Avoid taking liquorice.

**PMS-D**

- Add sources of phytoestrogens to the diet.
- Try taking wild yam (*Dioscorea villosa*) or black cohosh (*Cimicifuga racemosa*) as teas (both are made by decoction) or tinctures.

**PMS-P**

- Follow the advice for reducing oestrogen exposure and increasing phytoestrogens (*see* pages 205–8).
- Avoid animal fats in the diet.
- Supplement with vitamin B complex (containing 50mg per day of B6), magnesium, zinc and evening primrose oil.
- Select one or two herbs to relieve the kind of pain you are experiencing (*see* chapter 14).

Improving exercise, especially gentle exercise such as yoga, tai chi and walking, and learning relaxation and stress management techniques can help improve all forms of PMS. Partners and families can help by being aware of the 'time of the month' and exercising sensitivity to the woman's needs at that time.

## Enhancing Libido and Sexual Performance

Having a healthy sexual appetite and being able to participate fully in mutually satisfying sexual encounters is one of the great joys of life. Unfortunately, there are several factors which can interfere with this.

# Impotence

Strictly speaking, impotence refers to male sexual functions and describes the inability to attain and sustain an erection of the penis. Sometimes, the term 'impotence' is incorrectly used to describe an ability to attain an erection but an inability to ejaculate, an inability to sustain an erection due to premature ejaculation, or a decrease in the frequency with which an erection can be achieved. As men grow older it is common for them to find that they cannot achieve penetrative sex as often as they used to; likewise, it is common in long-term relationships for the initial flurry of intense sexual activity that occurs on beginning a relationship to settle into a less frequent pattern over time.

In cases of genuine impotence it is useful to see whether this occurs in conjunction with a decrease in libido. (Libido is discussed more fully opposite, but it refers to interest in sexual activity or the sexual appetite.) In men, if the libido is decreased then it is natural that erectile function is inhibited; this may improve as libido returns. If the libido is strong, but there is an impaired ability to achieve and maintain an erection, then this may indicate an underlying physical problem. Bear in mind that this distinction is not always reliable – an inability to relax and 'go with the flow' through being too self-conscious or worried about performance may frustrate the strongest ardour. Physical cause of impotence include:

- Arteriosclerosis (high cholesterol levels causing narrowing of the arteries),
- Heart disease,
- Diabetes,
- Low thyroid function.

If you do suffer from impotence, it is a good idea to have your cholesterol, blood sugar and thyroxine (thyroid hormone) levels checked.

By definition, not possessing a penis, women cannot suffer from impotence but they can still experience an impaired sexual response. In some women this manifests as an inability to relax the genital muscles and to produce lubricating vaginal secretions. This may often be because of hormonal changes associated with the menopause and may be helped by following the advice regarding menopause (*see* page 220), as well as by using lubricating creams and placing greater emphasis on non-penetrative sexual activities.

## Libido

It is quite normal for libido to vary over time and in response to changing physical, emotional and psychological circumstances such as tiredness, worry and stress. Also, many couples find that sexual appetite diminishes for a time after childbirth or when breast-feeding. Depression is another major cause of decreased libido and impotence, as are alcohol and drug abuse. If your sexual interest or activity is impaired by pain during intercourse, you should see a doctor to have this checked out. If sexual activity is complicated by previous bad experiences then working on this with an appropriately qualified psychotherapist can be of great help.

While there are many factors involved with achieving and maintaining optimum libido and sexual performance, there are several areas which should be looked at.

### Diet

As with all other areas of health it is important to have a good general diet to improve sexual performance. Alcohol intake should be kept at moderate levels or avoided completely, and drug use should be avoided. Sensory satisfaction from drug abuse can displace a healthy interest in sexual activity.

### Exercise

People often overlook the fact that sex is a physical activity. It is unreasonable to think that you can lead a sedentary life and then suddenly perform optimally in the bedroom (or wherever). Reasonable physical exercise outside of sexual activity can improve sexual appetite, stamina and enjoyment. Physical fitness improves sexual fitness.

## Relaxation

Being too uptight and tense can make it hard to let go and surrender to sexual passion. If your mind is on other things or your muscles are knotted up, you will not enjoy sex and neither will your partner. Managing stress and participating in relaxation activities such as yoga and meditation can be of help. Massage is a particularly useful relaxation technique – used for millennia by lovers as part of the sexual encounter. Make time for mutual massage, using aphrodisiac oils such as sandalwood (*Santalum album*) and rose (*Rosa damascena*).

## Happiness and self-esteem

People who feel good about themselves are more attractive to others and have an increased appetite and capacity for fulfilling sexual activity. Valuing yourself, caring about your self and trying to live a kind and respectful life with a positive and open attitude can help you achieve contentment and self-esteem. There are many self-help books and courses available that can help you find your own path to self-realisation. But make sure it is your own path, and not somebody else's.

## Familiarity

In long-term relationships, the novelty that provides a sexual thrill can often wear down. There are several books available giving advice on how to maintain the excitement in a relationship. It is important to be able to tell each other what you want from sex while respecting each others 'dos and don'ts'. Nurture each other with special times together other than sexual activity, such as meals, social events, baths and massage. One of the benefits of a long-term relationship is that you have the opportunity to explore your sexuality together.

## Herbs

There is a long tradition of using herbs as aphrodisiacs. Although some herbs promoted as a 'herbal viagra' may also overstimulate the circulation to the point that they cause high blood pressure, there are several much gentler herbs that can be very helpful in supporting sexual activity.

Strictly speaking, aphrodisiacs are herbs that stimulate sexual desire and they have been often used to bolster the declining sexual appetites and functions associated with the process of ageing, particularly in men. One of the most famous herbs from this perspective is the adaptogen Korean ginseng (*Panax ginseng*). It can indeed improve libido and sexual performance, but tends to be too strongly stimulating and can exacerbate high blood pressure and anxiety. All the same, the adaptogens as a group (*see* chapter 7) do have a major role to play in this area. My favourite adaptogens for enhancing sexual performance and desire are Siberian ginseng (*Eleutherococcus senticosus*) and ashwagandha (*Withania somnifera*). Many people are too tired and stressed to be able to gather the natural energies required to engage fully with the joys of sex. These two herbs improve physical stamina and endurance and help to achieve the sustained mental and emotional focus required in consistently satisfying sexual activity.

Few of the circulatory stimulants that have been employed for sexual purposes are appropriate; often the relaxing and calming herbs that strengthen the nervous system (*see* chapter 14) are more appropriate and give more benefits. Gingko (*Gingko biloba*) is an exception. This herb improves general circulation and may improve sexual performance.

Saw palmetto (*Serenoa serulata*) has long been considered as a sexual tonic herb for men and this may be partially due to its effects in relieving benign prostatic hyperplasia – a condition causing enlargement of the prostate gland. Damiana (*Turnera diffusa*) was formerly so renowned as a sexual tonic herb that its older botanical name was *Turnera aphrodisiaca*. There is a small amount of research supporting its reputation in enhancing libido, erectile function and improvements in fertility in men.

One of the most interesting of the aphrodisiac herbs is a South American shrub called muira puama (*Ptychopetalum olacoides*), also known as 'potency wood'. It has long been taken in South American countries for impotence and sexual fatigue, and as a tonic for the nervous system.

Many foods have a reputation as aphrodisiacs, including garlic. Garlic may be of benefit if both people involved in sexual activity consume it – that way the smell tends not to be noticed. Garlic's reputation as a promoter of sexual performance may rely in part on its cholesterol-lowering activities, especially for men.

Although many aphrodisiacs are not specified for female use, this may reflect longstanding gender bias. It is not widely appreciated that testosterone plays an important role in female as well as male sexual function, so that many of the purportedly male aphrodisiacs may also enhance female sexual appetite and performance.

## Supporting Fertility

It is essential to have any fertility problems explored fully by your medical practitioner. The following advice can be of general benefit to all women and men preparing to start a family.

### Women

- Try and achieve your ideal weight – being overweight or underweight can affect fertility levels. Exercise to this end should not be excessive because women who exercise too much have experienced fertility problems.
- Following a balanced healthy diet is vital. Keep the intake of caffeine and alcohol low and increase the consumption of foods containing vitamins B12 and E, as well as iron and zinc. It is important to supplement the diet with folic acid around the time leading up to conception and in early pregnancy to help prevent birth defects of the nervous system (such as spina bifida) and cleft palate.
- It can be helpful to follow a detox regime (see chapter 5) to cleanse the body before beginning to conceive.

- Chasteberry (*Vitex agnus-castus*) can sometimes be of benefit in regulating the periods before conception and in improving ovulation if there is a problem in this respect.

## Men

- Try and achieve a healthy weight.

- Follow a good diet that is low in saturated fat, alcohol, and refined and processed foods and sugar. The diet should be rich in fruit, vegetables and protein sources such as grains and pulses. Vitamin C and zinc supplements can aid male fertility. A good source of zinc is pumpkin seeds – eat enough pumpkin seeds to cover your palm each day. Zinc improves testosterone and sperm production and motility. Selenium is also essential for male fertility – eating just one Brazil nut per day can provide an excellent selenium supplement.

- The testicles should be kept cooler than the rest of the body. Avoid tight underwear and trousers, and use light, cool fabrics such as cotton and linen.

- Oestrogens in cow's milk can cause adverse effects on male fertility, so dairy milk should be kept to a minimum or avoided when trying to conceive.

- The herb saw palmetto (*Serenoa serulata*) may be of value in improving male fertility.

## Pregnancy

Support for women and their babies in pregnancy is too wide a subject to discuss in detail here. However, the need for increased nutritional intake and for rest should be recognised. Be wary of taking herbs during pregnancy unless on the advice of a herbal practitioner.

One herb that can be considered generally safe and useful is raspberry leaf (*Rubus idaeus*). This has a reputation for helping to prepare the body for birth, facilitating an easy delivery and helping the uterus return quickly to its pre-pregnant state after birth. I can vouch for these benefits from my own clinical experience. Research shows that raspberry leaves possess constituents which can both relax and stimulate, and these actions appear to be able to vary as required by the body, so ensuring appropriate uterine activity at all stages of pregnancy, birth and recovery. It is best to begin taking raspberry leaf tea as an infusion at a dose of 2–8g per day from 12 weeks before the due date and continuing for 8–12 weeks after the birth.

## Breast-feeding

As well as having potential health benefits for the mother (there is a possible protective effect against breast cancer), breast-feeding certainly has major benefits for the child.

A number of herbs have excellent traditional reputations for improving breast milk production in lactating women, including vervain (*Verbena officinalis*) and borage (*Borago officinalis*).

When breast-feeding there is an increase of 50–100% in the need for dietary nutrients. Of particular importance are calcium and magnesium, essential fatty acids (GLA and omega-3 EFAs are vital for the development of the baby's nervous system), protein, vitamins B, C and E, zinc, selenium and folic acid. Seaweed is a good source of iodine to support the thyroid gland.

## The Menopause

The menopause refers to the time when a woman's periods cease. The perimenopause refers to the years just before and just after the periods cease, during which changes may be experienced reflecting hormonal adjustments inside the body. The perimenopause can vary in length, but typically lasts from around the ages of 45–55, with the menopause itself occurring at about the age of 50. The age at which a woman's mother experienced menopause may her give an indication of when she might be likely to expect her own.

Many of the changes experienced around the menopause are associated with a fall in oestrogen levels. These include changes in the length and regularity of the menstrual cycle and its flow, hot flushes, sweats at night, vaginal dryness, skin and hair changes, mood disturbances (including tearfulness and confusion) and fatigue. Not all women experience all of these changes and some women pass through the menopause noticing very few changes at all. After the menopause, the reduction in oestrogen gradually exposes women to the same risk of heart disease as men, as well as increasing the risk of osteoporosis, especially if there is a family history of this condition.

Recently, there has been much attention on the negative aspects of the menopause and it has been presented as an illness – specifically as a deficiency disease of oestrogen. It is more helpful to view the meno-pause as a normal and natural process that can generally be managed gently and left to progress to its conclusion – just like pregnancy.

Having a positive attitude towards the menopause is desirable, but this may be harder for some women than others, and those who have been unable to have children may not wish to celebrate the ending of their reproductive years. For women with grown-up children the menopause can represent a rite of passage from child-bearing years to those where there is more time to focus on their own needs, interests and desires. The following advice can help to ease the transition through this important phase:

- Learn how to protect against heart disease after the menopause (*see* chapter 10). It is important to decrease saturated and hydrogenated fats and to increase monounsaturated and polyunsaturated fats because, as oestrogen decreases, the levels of 'good' (HDL) cholesterol also decrease and those of 'bad' (LDL) cholesterol rise.
- Take steps to prevent osteoporosis (*see* chapter 12) and be careful to eat foods rich in calcium and magnesium, and avoid foods high in phosphorus (such as red meat, processed foods and cola drinks) as these reduce the levels of minerals in the bones.

- Vitamin E taken at a dose of 400mg per day can reduce hot flushes; vitamin E cream can be very good applied to the vagina to reduce dryness.

- Phytoestrogens in the diet can modulate sharp fluctuations in oestrogen levels, so reducing menopausal symptoms and possibly helping to prevent heart disease and osteoporosis.

- Phytoestrogen herbs such as black cohosh (*Cimicifuga racemosa*) can help prevent or reduce hot flushes and vaginal dryness, and stabilise the body generally during the menopause.

## Hormone replacement therapy (HRT)

Conventional medicine offers hormone replacement therapy (HRT) as a treatment for the symptoms of the menopause. In my view, HRT only seems a suitable option for women who experience severe symptoms of menopausal changes or who are at high risk of developing osteoporosis, but it is inappropriate for most women. Apart from suggesting that there is something fundamentally 'wrong' with the menopause, some women do not react to HRT very well and their symptoms can worsen, or they can feel unwell when taking it.

There are some concerns about the use of HRT increasing the risk of breast and uterine (endometrial) cancers. Additionally, HRT is only a temporary solution and any benefits are soon lost after stopping taking it. In some women, HRT does no more than delay the full force of menopausal symptoms when they stop taking HRT, sometimes ten years after they would normally have gone through this process.

### The hormone therapies

The type of HRT preparation is important. Oestrogen reduces the risk of heart disease but when HRT is combined oestrogen and prog-esterone this beneficial effect is negated. However, when only oestrogen is taken there is an increased risk of breast and uterine cancers. New HRT drugs known as SERMs (selective estrogen receptor modulators) are now being developed which should provide safer treatment options as they aim to supply oestrogen only to tissues that can benefit from it (the bones and cardiovascular system).

## 'Natural progesterone'
This is often marketed as containing wild yam (*Dioscorea villosa*) and the implication is that this is a herbal product. However, wild yam does not contain progesterone, nor is it likely that the body can convert the constituents of wild yam into progesterone, but it is possible to convert a chemical contained in wild yams (dioscin) into progesterone. Most natural progesterone products contain this laboratory-derived hormone, a type of synthetic conventional HRT, and it should only be considered and prescribed by medically qualified doctors

## The male menopause
Men continue to be capable of fathering a child long after women cease to be able to conceive. There is no dramatic change in the hormones in men directly equivalent to the fall in oestrogen in women, but testosterone levels do gradually decrease in men as they age. This may have more significant effects for some men than others. As testosterone levels drop, so does sexual activity, and although there are wide variations, most men start to experience a decline in sexual functions between their late 40s and late 50s. This time of transition may be accompanied by changes in mood and outlook corresponding to women's menopausal experiences, at least as regards psychological changes.

Symptoms of a pronounced 'male menopause' similar to those encountered in women, including hot flushes, have been reported. Given that the male reproductive system is less complex than that of the female, it is to be expected that hormonal changes will be less dramatic, but they do still occur and need to be treated with respect and consideration. The traditional male tonic herbs such as saw palmetto (*Serenoa serulata*) and damiana (*Turnera diffusa*) have a potential role to play in helping men to cope with hormonal changes in later years.

# Cancers

## Prostate cancer

In men, prostate cancer is the most commonly diagnosed reproductive-system cancer in the West. Antioxidant flavonoids (*see* chapter 6) may help prevent it, as well as regular intake of phytoestrogens from soya products and other foods. There is good evidence that a reduction in consumption of saturated fat and refined carbohydrates, together with optimal intake of vitamins D and E and selenium, can decrease your risk of developing prostate cancer.

## Breast cancer

Breast cancer is the most common cancer in women. There is a significant hereditary component to this type of cancer and if your mother or sister has had it then you should be ensure you take preventive action by:

- Reducing exposure to oestrogen (*see* page 205);
- Decreasing saturated fat intake;
- Increasing soluble fibre intake;
- Eating plenty of antioxidant sources. Eating plenty of vegetables that interfere with oestrogen metabolism (such as cabbage, broccoli and cauliflower);
- Eating plenty of phytoestrogens;
- Avoiding obesity;
- Keeping alcohol consumption to a low level.

## Cervical cancer

It is important to have cervical smears regularly to detect cervical dysplasia (pre-cancerous changes to the cervix), thus improving the chances of detecting any potential development of cervical cancer at an early stage. To help prevent cancer of the cervix, it is important to:

- Maintain a high intake of antioxidants;
- Keep saturated fat levels low;
- Stop smoking – women who smoke are three times more likely to have cervical changes than those who do not.

# Herbs for the Reproductive System

## Black cohosh

Black cohosh (*Cimicifuga racemosa*) is a North American plant that is particularly useful for reducing symptoms of hot flushes and vaginal dryness during the menopause. It represents a natural alternative to HRT if these are your primary symptoms. It is also used to treat arthritis and rheumatism and is particularly helpful for women who experience these kinds of problems during the menopause. The roots are used medically and they should be taken as a decoction at a dose of 0.5–1.0g per cup, repeated 3 times a day. This plant is becoming an endangered species and so you should make sure that you obtain only guaranteed sustainable products.

## Chasteberry

The benefits of chasteberry (*Vitex agnus-castus*) and how to take it are described on page 227.

## Dong quai

Dong quai (*Angelica sinensis*) has been called 'women's ginseng' because of its reputation for improving reproductive health in females. I discourage the use of this term because neither is this plant in the ginseng family, nor can it be used for general purposes by all women – specifically, it should be avoided if you suffer from heavy periods.

However, dong quai does possess many excellent benefits for women. It contains beta-sitosterol, which lowers cholesterol, and it can also lower blood pressure; these two qualities can help prevent heart disease in post-menopausal women. This herb can improve the length of the menstrual cycle if you have a long cycle with weak flow. It is also very good for preventing period pain and as a supportive herb to take after pregnancy and while breast-feeding. Some studies have suggested it may improve female fertility. The root is the part of the plant used and this should be taken as tea made by decoction at a dose of 1–3g per cup, repeated 3 times a day.

## Damiana

Damiana (*Turnera diffusa*) is considered to be a tonic herb for the reproductive system in men and women. It is particularly valued as a herb for treating sexual fatigue, impotence and lowered libido, as well as for general nervous exhaustion. The leaves are used as a tea or tincture. The tea should be prepared by infusion at a dose of 2–4g of the leaves per day. Occasionally, the resins from the plant can cause mild stomach irritation – to offset this effect it is best to drink the tea after meals.

## Linseeds

Linseeds (*Linum usitatissimum*) contain phytoestrogenic lignans; in addition they contain soluble fibre (which helps them to reduce cholesterol levels) and omega-3 essential fatty acids. This combination of properties means that linseeds can be taken as a general phytoestrogen to treat conditions of oestrogen excess and to protect the heart following the menopause. Take 2 teaspoons to 1 dessertspoon of the raw whole (not dehulled) seeds each morning with water. You can take the seeds sprinkled on your breakfast cereal and eaten or mixed in a cup of water or juice and drunk. Whichever method you use, it is very important that you wash the seeds down with 2 further glasses of water.

## Muira puama

The bark and roots of this South American tree (*Ptychopetalum olacoides*) have traditionally been employed as an aphrodisiac to increase sexual desire and improve the ability to gain and maintain an erection. The active constituents in the plant are not very water soluble and the bark or roots need to be decocted (simmered) for 20–60 minutes to achieve an adequate extraction. For this reason it is best to take this herb as a tincture at a dose of 3ml per day of the 1:2 tincture, taken in water.

## Saw palmetto

The benefits of saw palmetto, *Serenoa serulata*, and how to take it are described on page 228.

### KEY HERB FOR THE FEMALE REPRODUCTIVE SYSTEM

## CHASTEBERRY

**Scientific name** *Vitex agnus-castus*

**Plant family** Verbenaceae (Verbena family)

**Type of plant** A shrub or small tree.

**Part used** The fruits (berries).

**Phytochemicals** Flavonoids, iridoid glycosides, volatile oil.

**Actions** Galactagogue; menstrual regulator.

**Indications** Vitex can be used to normalise irregular, long or short menstrual cycles, and to relieve most types of premenstrual syndrome (apart from that which is predominantly PMS-C – the sugar cravings type) and period pain that is preceded by PMS. It is a supportive herb in the treatment of some cases of infertility (where progesterone levels are low or prolactin levels are high) and improves milk flow when breast-feeding. It is also useful for conditions of oestrogen excess, such as fibroids and endometriosis.

**Preparations** Best taken as a tincture. The 1:1 strength tincture is taken at a dose of 5–20 drops per day in the morning with water.

**Combinations** Chasteberry is usually taken on its own.

**Cautions** Avoid taking in cases of period pain that occur without preceding PMS. It is wise to avoid taking this herb at the same time as any conventional reproductive hormonal medication (such as HRT, IVF and the pill) unless on the advice of a herbal practitioner. Avoid during pregnancy.

**Conservation** Chasteberry is a relatively common Mediterranean plant and is not considered to be endangered.

## KEY HERB FOR THE MALE REPRODUCTIVE SYSTEM

# SAW PALMETTO

**Scientific name** *Serenoa serulata*

**Plant family** Arecaceae (Palm family)

**Type of plant** A shrub palm native to south-east North America.

**Part used** Fruits (berries).

**Phytochemicals** Flavonoids, lipids, phytosterols, polysaccharides.

**Actions** Anti-inflammatory, antispasmodic, modulates male hormone levels.

**Indications** To support male sexual functions from middle age onwards. Preventing and treating benign prostatic hypertrophy (a common condition involving enlargement of the prostate gland and leading to impairment of urination and discomfort). It is also used for prostatitis (inflammation of the prostate gland).

**Preparations** A decoction of the berries taken at a dose of 2–4g of the dried berries per day. The 1:2 tincture (made with high alcohol levels the better to extract the active constituents) can be taken at a dose of 2–4ml per day in water.

**Combinations** Saw palmetto combines well with nettle roots in the treatment of benign prostatic hypertrophy. Use 2g of each herb per day as a tea made by decoction.

**Cautions** This plant is considered to be safe and is well tolerated in most circumstances.

**Conservation** There are no concerns about the environmental status of this plant.

# Chapter 14

# HERBS FOR THE MIND & EMOTIONS –

## Becoming balanced and content, and improving your mental power

Our thoughts and feelings can have profound effects on the body – for example, anxiety can impact on the digestive system and mental stress can cause muscular tension. If we are able to achieve and maintain a positive mental focus and a balanced emotional state then beneficial effects will follow for the body as a whole. Good mental and emotional health helps to foster good physical health. One of the great strengths of herbal medicine is its ability to improve the activities of the nervous system. Herbs that are particularly helpful in this regard are described as 'nervines'.

The emotional body is where we experience fear, anxiety, sorrow, and all the other feelings that can affect our well-being. There are several herbs that are able to soothe and heal our emotions and help us to feel excitement, hope, contentment and joy. The mental body is where we reflect, organise, plan, predict and create, and its activities may also be enhanced by herbal medicines.

The nervous system extends throughout the entire body and it comprises the central nervous system (the brain and spinal cord) and the peripheral nervous system (the nerves that branch off from the spinal cord to the furthest reaches of the human body). It enables our movement (through the nervous supply to muscles), experience of physical sensation (the five senses plus specialised sensing of temperature, vibration, etc.), emotional responses and thoughts.

# The Mind and the Emotions

The distinctions between the mind and emotions may not be as clear-cut as they first seem. Traditionally, the two aspects were seen as so separate that we still talk of 'thinking with the head and feeling with the heart'. In fact, we clearly understand that thought lies in the brain, but the emotions have a much vaguer place of residence – they seem to pervade us, filling out our whole body and even spreading out beyond us to touch others. We may say that 'I could feel her anger as soon as I entered the room', or that 'the tension was palpable'. In general, we tend to see the mind as contained and precisely located, and as a calculating and controlling entity, whereas we see our emotional nature as being free, widely pervading and running easily out of control.

We view our minds as objective, rational, logical, cold and abstracted, and our emotions as subjective, intuitive, responsive, hot and engaging, but in reality there are many areas of overlap. Intellectual reflection can lead to emotional responses and emotional responses can in turn be interpreted and adapted by the mind. It is interesting how we make value judgements about people depending on their individual mind–emotion balance; for example, we frequently express distaste for the heavily intellectual person who we may consider to be arrogant, lacking in humanity, and all in all 'a bit of a cold fish'. Similarly, we may consider someone who is too emotional to be unstable and too intense; we might advise them that they need to 'get things into perspective' – a key ability of the reflective intellect.

There is a spectrum of activity that ranges from the purely emotional state to the purely intellectual. As with most things it is usually best to avoid extremes and to focus ourselves in the middle of the spectrum. It is natural that we will oscillate now and again, but if we spend too much time at either extreme we will probably miss out on many of life's worthwhile experiences. The goal then is to balance and integrate our mind and emotions.

# Maintaining a Healthy Nervous System

We all have the potential to function on four interrelated levels:

- Physical,
- Emotional,
- Mental,
- Spiritual.

The emotional and mental levels are the central ones, capable of connecting the spiritual and the physical aspects of our being. Sometimes we are prone to having our energies focused on one or other of these levels. While none of the levels is 'better' than any other, there is a general line of progression – from a mainly physical, material existence, reliant on the attainment of possessions, to a spiritual life where satisfaction is gained from significant actions and experiences.

Many of us are still at the stage of trying to achieve the right balance between emotional and mental well-being. The overall goal is to achieve a positive and harmonious emotional body combined with mental strength, clarity and power. With the constant demands and strains on our nervous system, this sometimes seems an impossible goal to attain. However, there are some basic strategies that we can follow to help us to this end.

## Avoiding mental and emotional fatigue

It is hard to focus on improving our mental and emotional capabilities when they are so depleted that basic survival seems the only option. To ease the pressure and open up the potential for energy to accumulate, it is necessary to address the 'brain drains' represented by stress, overwork, hyperactivity, emotional insecurity and emotional extremism, each of which can lead to a state of nervous exhaustion.

The first stage is to step back and look at our mental and emotional expenditure. Where do we expend our nervous energy?

Are we using it efficiently? It may be of benefit to talk over your particular situation with a counsellor or psychotherapist. There are also a number of good books and courses that deal with stress and time management, and these may help you with the sort of positive changes you need to make in your life.

## Thinking positively

Much has been written about the 'power of positive thinking', to the point where it has become a cliché. While it is true that positive thinking is worth little unless it is followed by positive action, the fact remains that a positive attitude, in both mental and emotional terms, is a genuinely potent life force.

Positive, in these terms, does not mean unrealistic but working productively with our own individual realities. Remember the phrase 'energy follows thought' and constantly remind yourself of it. In effect, if we are always thinking that a negative outcome will happen then it probably will, but if we focus on positive outcomes then they become more likely. We do this by visualising the goal we want to achieve and then setting towards it while remaining open to learning from experience along the way, feeling good levels of self-esteem about ourselves and focusing on the positive results that we encounter.

## Meditation

Meditation may be the most powerful way of engendering a positive approach to life. By using meditation it is possible to visualise goals, reflect on options and experiences, and gain insights into our life situation. There are numerous books and courses dealing with the many approaches to meditation. It is worth taking time to find one that chimes with you. Meditation is quintessentially a simple yet powerful technique that with continued practice accumulates its positive effects. By setting aside just ten minutes a day, you can quickly reap enormous benefits.

## Exercise and relaxation

Physical exercise is important for the functioning of the brain since it needs a high blood flow to meet the heavy demands of the brain cells for nutrition and oxygen supply. Exerting the body also helps to relax the mind and emotions – participating in (or even just watching!) competitive sport can provide a great emotional release.

It is important to remember that the mind and emotions need stimulating as well as the body. This can be achieved by a variety of means, including pastimes, hobbies and social activities such as:

- Intellectual games and puzzles, for example crosswords, bridge and chess;
- Social intercourse, conversation and debate;
- Theatre, music, visual arts, literature and dance.

## Diet

As in all the systems we have looked at, the correct balanced diet is vital. In terms of the nervous system, the following advice will be helpful.

- The diet should be low in saturated fat and in line with the advice given on the cardiovascular system (*see* Chapter 10) to avoid arteriosclerosis developing in the arteries of the brain and to minimise the risk of having a stroke (a bleed into the brain).
- Alcohol damages the brain cells and should be consumed in moderation only.
- Antioxidants can help protect the brain cells from damage by free radicals.
- The brain cells have a high demand for the B complex vitamins; ensuring an adequate supply of these may help to enhance brain functions and protect the brain from future degenerative disease (such as dementia).
- The brain cells need a good supply of essential fatty acids (omega-6 and omega-3), so it helps to supplement daily with an oil such as hemp oil (1 teaspoon a day).

- Brain activity can be disrupted and fatigued by blood sugar fluctuations so avoid overloading the brain with sugary foods and refined carbohydrates.

- Acetylcholine is one of the major neurotransmitters in the brain. Its activities can be supported by ensuring that the diet contains sources of choline, such as apples, bananas, oranges, cauliflower, whole grains and nuts.

## The power of sleep

The nervous system becomes strained without adequate sleep. During sleep the body has an opportunity to replenish energy and to repair daily neurological wear and tear. It is important to have good-quality, nourishing deep sleep. When we are anxious or worried, sleep becomes fragile because the mind tends to become overwhelmed by circular thoughts and fear.

Sleep requirements vary between individuals and between phases of life, but around eight hours a night is a good rule of thumb. Some people are 'night owls' while others are 'early birds', but there seem to be distinct advantages in getting to bed earlier! Several of the herbs mentioned later on in this chapter (*see* pages 239–50) can help promote a healthy sleeping pattern.

## Breathe deep

The most efficient way to fulfil our brain's high oxygen requirements is to adopt a proper deep-breathing pattern. Anxiety states are associated with shallow breathing and a consequent lack of oxygen supply to the brain. It is good policy to check how you are breathing occasionally – if you are feeling stressed or anxious, the chances are that your breathing will be shallow. A good technique to improve your breathing is to place a hand over your abdomen and then try to breathe 'into your hand'. You do this by breathing right down into the abdomen so that you make it move visibly in and out. An even simpler technique is just to breathe with your mouth slightly open – this will automatically make you breathe a little deeper.

# Herbs and the Nervous System

The herbs that have positive influences on the nervous system are known as 'nervines'. Traditionally, herbs in this category have been said to 'strengthen the nerves' or 'comfort the brain'. Nervines work with the nervous system in a non-aggressive way, gently supporting and influencing without unduly impairing our mental and emotional faculties, leaving us in control.

While conventional medicine focuses on conditions such as clinical depression and Alzheimer's disease, the herbal approach is to look at strengthening or balancing the emotional or mental state. There are herbs that can help with feelings of sadness, anxiety, anger and fear, as well as with mental problems such as poor concentration, lack of focus and poor memory. Nervines also have a part to play in helping the physical body deal with the effects of stress, pressure and nervous tension.

The key drugs used by conventional medicine for treating the nervous system are antidepressants, anxiolytics (drugs that reduce anxiety states), sedatives, antipsychotics and painkillers. While some of these drugs are essential in the initial treatment of extreme pathological conditions, they are all very strong in their action, several are addictive and they all tend to suppress or take over normal functions. Herbs can offer valuable alternatives in treating some of these conditions.

*Caution*
If you are taking conventional drugs to treat a nervous-system disorder, you should not take nervine herbs, either as replacement for or supplementary to conventional medication, without discussing the issue with your doctor and a herbal practitioner.

## The actions of the nervines

Just as conventional drugs can be classified into groups depending on their activity, nervine herbs can be classified into groups such as antidepressants, anxiolytics, sedatives, hypnotics (herbs that aid sleep), nervous trophorestoratives (herbs that nourish a depleted nervous system) and mental relaxants (herbs that ease mental tension). In addition, the adaptogens (*see* chapter 7) are important nervines as they have the ability to improve mental performance and modulate the body's response to stress.

## Dosage

The dosage at which many of the herbal nervines are taken can be critical, especially with those that have anxiolytic, sedative or hypnotic activities. These three actions are interrelated and many herbs that have one of these actions will also tend to have the others depending on the dosage. For instance, a herb that has an anxiolytic action at a small dose may have sedative effects at a higher dose and hypnotic effects at a yet higher dose. So, limeflowers (*Tilia* species) which are mildly anxiolytic at a dose of around 2 teaspoons to a cup, are sedative at double that dose and hypnotic at triple the dose.

In this book, the lower dosage ranges are given because we are seeking to protect gently, to modulate and enhance nervous activity, rather than to achieve a stronger impact. Many herbs can achieve profound effects on the nervous system by taking the edge off nervous disruption and the associated agitation, helping to put a brake on the escalation of nervous stress.

## Benefits

Taking appropriate nervine herbs, in conjunction with adjustments to lifestyle, can bring major benefits for our emotional and mental well-being. Emotionally we can become:

- Calmer;
- More content;
- Able to access positive emotions as well as dealing with negative ones;
- More in touch with our emotions and open to exploring them.

Overall, this helps us to become more rounded individuals who feel self-confident and self-assured. Mentally we can gain:

- Better focus;
- More control, with enhanced concentration and memory;
- The ability to deal with stress;
- Improved levels of imaginative and creative activity.

As organised and decisive individuals we are able to pursue our own destinies, achieve worthwhile goals and be of service to others.

# Herbs for the Mind and Emotions

The actions of many of the nervines are very similar and it can be hard to pinpoint the differences that lie between them. It often comes down to a subjective sense of the particular qualities and affinities that these herbs seem to possess. Where appropriate I have included some of my own subjective impressions based on working with these plants over the years. These impressions may strike a chord with you about your own emotional and mental state and guide you towards the herbs that might best suit you.

## Circulatory stimulants

Several herbs help to improve the blood supply to the brain, including ginger (*Zingiber officinale*), ginkgo (*Gingko biloba*) and rosemary (*Rosmarinus officinalis*) (*see* chapter 10). To this group we can add sage (*Salvia officinalis*) and the leaves of the lesser periwinkle (*Vinca minor*). Herbs that enhance brain circulation can improve:

- Concentration;
- Mental focus;
- Decision making;
- Mental energy and alertness;
- Memory function.

It is worth considering using circulatory stimulants at times when your brain is having to cope with increased demands, for example when revising for exams or researching for a project or presentation. They are also of general value in supporting mental functions, and some may help to prevent or slow down the progression of dementia. The most suitable herbs to use for this are rosemary and ginkgo (*see* chapter 10).

## Adaptogens

Many of these have an ability to improve mental performance and to protect the body from the adverse effects of stress (*see* chapter 7). They also tend to engender mental energy and creativity, as well as supporting a positive attitude towards the challenges of life. My two favourite nervine adaptogens are ashwagandha (*Withania somnifera*) and Siberian ginseng (*Eleutherococcus senticosus*) – these are non-stimulating and suit modern lifestyles well. Ashwagandha has proven useful in the treatment of depression and is one of the most valuable adaptogens for this condition. It is also suitable for use where there is overexcitement and an inability to calm down.

# Chamomile

Chamomile (*Matricaria recutita*) was our key herb for the digestive system (*see* chapter 9). It is particularly useful when nervous tension causes upset digestion and it is often useful in irritable bowel syndrome. Although a well-known and widely used beverage, the healing power of a cup of good-quality chamomile tea should not be underestimated. Sipped slowly while hot, chamomile tea has a gently calming and relaxing effect. It can even help relieve mild pain, such as period pain and tension headaches. Chamomile is one of the best nervine herbs for long-term general use.

# Kava

Kava (*Piper methysticum*) helps to reduce feelings of anxiety as well as being an excellent antispasmodic for muscular pain and tension (*see* chapter 12). Kava is indeed a 'tranquilliser' in the best sense of the word; it will help to promote peace and tranquillity for those suffering from feelings of fear, agitation and insecurity. It is, however, currently a banned substance in the UK as explained in Chapter 12.

## Borage

The sixteenth-century herbalist John Gerard wrote that borage flowers are used 'for the comfort of the heart, for the driving away of sorrow and increasing the joy of the minde'. There is also an old verse that proclaims that 'I, borage, bring always courage'. The pale blue flowers of borage (*Borago officinalis*) remain highly praised for their inspirational beauty and the leaves are still taken as a herbal remedy. Borage is considered a nervous trophorestorative, a nerve tonic with nourishing and supportive effects for the nervous tissues. It is a herb that can be helpful in treating nervous exhaustion and emotional depletion leading to a state of feeling flat and unmotivated. It is a good herb for supporting the mood during periods of convalescence and physical weakness. I favour using borage where energy levels are low and the emotions seem to be drained, worn out or confused.

Borage has lovely, cheering flowers and is very easy to grow. A tea can be made from the fresh flowers in summer – use half a dozen flowers infused in a cup of water, or the flowers can be added to salads. You can also freeze the flowers in ice cubes for use later in the year. To make borage tea from dried herbs, use 2 teaspoons of the dried flowers and leaves and prepare by infusion. Drink 2–3 cups a day.

## Californian poppy

This member of the poppy family (*Papaveraceae*), with delicate orange flowers, is another easy-to-grow and attractive plant that

will enhance any garden. It is the state flower of California and
was formerly used by several Native American tribes as a mild
painkiller and hypnotic. Poppies are the source of the potent
painkiller morphine and related opioid analgesics. The
Californian poppy (*Eschscholzia californica*) has a gentle and non-
addictive action but can be of value as a mild painkiller for
chronic pain such as recurrent tension headaches, helping to
reduce the sensation of pain and lessen its debilitating effects. It
is also useful if you are prone to being hyperactive or to feelings
of restlessness and irritability.

Californian poppy tea is prepared from the dried aerial parts of
the plant (leaves, stem and flowers) by infusion. Use 2–3
teaspoons of the dried herb to a cup and take up to 3 cups a day.

## Feverfew

Feverfew (*Tanacetum parthenium*) is a pain-relieving herb for the
nervous system. It is used specifically for migraine headaches. In
order to reap the rewards of this plant it is necessary to take it in
the correct way and for a sufficient period of time. The herb
works best when taken fresh, not dried. A tincture made from
the fresh plant is the best preparation and 1ml (of the 1:3
tincture) should be taken in water each morning. Alternatively,
if you grow feverfew, eat one fresh leaf of the plant each day
when in season. If you do this, it is important to chop the leaf
finely and combine it with a sandwich or other food – contact of
the neat herb with the mouth can cause mouth ulcers. It is
necessary to continue taking feverfew daily (it is taken to
prevent migraine attacks, not to treat them when they arrive)
for at least 6 months. I have seen excellent results with this herb
but the time it takes to build up its effects can be substantial.

Many migraine sufferers have a chronic habituation to
conventional painkillers and it is necessary to come off these

before the nervous system is able to repair itself and deal with the migraine naturally. If you are dependent on painkillers, you are advised to consult a herbalist to help you withdraw from your medication.

## Hops

The flower heads (strobiles) of the hop vine (*Humulus lupulus*) have long been used in brewing beer; they also have a long history as a herbal medicine. Taken as a herbal tea, hops have sedative and sleep-inducing qualities. They can be useful in helping us to deal with brief periods of sleeplessness and agitation, but should only be used for short periods of time (1–2 weeks at a time). Hops are suitable for use when we experience an overstimulation of energy such that it becomes hard for us to 'switch off'. This can happen when overexcitement makes us so hyped up that we become unable to relax and settle down, interfering with our ability to enjoy the moment. Occasional use of hops for episodes of difficulty in falling asleep can be of great benefit. Hops are also useful for the kind of situation where we might say 'I'm too tired to go to sleep' – the hops interfere in the pattern of exhaustion and resulting nervous disruption.

Hop tea is made by infusing 3 or 4 whole flower heads and drinking a cup in the daytime to calm states of hyperactivity and nervous agitation, or before going to bed if you want to use it to help you sleep. It is somewhat bitter to taste, but an excellent way of overcoming this is to add one teaspoon of chamomile to the hops; this makes a much more pleasant drink, which is also more effective than hops taken alone.

## Lavender

Although we may think of lavender (*Lavandula officinalis*) as merely a pleasant, mildly relaxing scent, in fact it is quite a strong sedative when taken as a herbal tea or tincture. It has similar indications as for hops (to calm hyperactivity states and induce sleep), but has a more pronounced influence on muscular relaxation so that it can also be taken to ease states of nervous tension that result in tense muscles.

Lavender tea has a 'perfume' that is not to everyone's taste and it may be easier to take this herb as a tincture. For a sedative effect, 2–5ml of the 1:2 tincture can be taken each day. For a hypnotic action to promote sleep, a single dose of 5–8ml of the tincture should be taken in a little water on going to bed. As a tea, lavender is prepared by infusion; it combines well with hops and the bitterness of these counterbalances the perfumed sweetness of the lavender flowers. A teaspoon of lavender flowers can be combined with 2 hop flower heads for each cup. A traditional sleeping pillow made by filling a muslin bag with equal parts of lavender and hops, laid at the side of your normal pillow in bed, can be very helpful in improving your sleeping pattern.

## Lemon balm

Lemon balm (*Melissa officinalis*) is one of the easiest herbs to grow – to the point that it may be considered a weed. For all that, it grows so well that the volatile oil distilled from this plant is one of the finest, and the most expensive, of all the plant oils. (It is expensive because, as with roses, it takes huge amounts of the fresh plant to produce a small amount of the pure oil.) It is called lemon balm because of the lemony smell of the oil. The leaves are used in herbal medicine to make a tea that is amongst the most delicious and refreshing of all beverages.

Lemon balm elevates the mood and helps to relieve feelings of despondency and despair, replacing them with those of optimism. This plant opens the heavy velvet curtains that sometimes shroud the human spirit and lets in the light. It is a herb that can help to pierce the gloom during those times when we find it hard to see the purpose and meaning in life, finding it difficult to take the next step. In the seventeenth century, diarist and horticulturalist John Evelyn wrote that lemon balm 'is sovereign for the brain, strengthening the memory and driving away melancholy'. The traditional reputation that lemon balm has for improving memory is yet to be proven but it may reflect an enhancement of circulation to the brain. In addition to its antidepressant action, lemon balm is a relaxant, and antispasmodic, antioxidant and antiviral. This broad spectrum of actions, combined with its safety and great taste, make lemon balm one of the best herbal teas to take on a regular basis.

The tea is made by infusing 2 teaspoons of the dried leaves or a small handful of chopped fresh leaves. It is important to place a cover on the tea while it is brewing in order to prevent loss of the volatile oil. This really is a tea to savour. You can drink 3–4 cups a day and it will help to relax you and prepare you for sleep when taken in the evenings.

## Limeflowers

Limeflowers (*Tilia* species) provide another very enjoyable herbal tea. 'Limeflowers' are actually made up of the small flowers themselves combined with the leaf-like structures (bracts) attached to them. Limeflowers are slightly sedative and can help improve sleep. As a calming herb they have a particular affinity for the heart and blood vessels and are sometimes considered to be a 'cardiac sedative'. They are particularly useful to take if you suffer from angina, high blood pressure or high cholesterol levels, and if anxiety states are accompanied by palpitations. In addition, they are settling to jangled nerves and help to reduce feelings of anger and aggression. Limeflower tea is also physically soothing to the throat and lungs due to the mucilage that the flowers contain.

Limeflower tea, also known as linden tea, is made by infusing 2 teaspoons of the flowers and bracts. The tea can be taken 3–4 times a day and will aid sleep when taken at bedtime. It has a satisfying honeyed taste and is particularly suitable if you tend to find herbal teas too bitter tasting.

## Oats

As a food, oats (*Avena sativa*) are an excellent source of vitamins and minerals. The nutritive value of oats is best gained by eating them in porridge or muesli each morning. Oat bran is an excellent source of soluble fibre and can be consumed regularly to help control cholesterol levels. Herbalists use oatstraw for the nervous system as a tonic and trophorestorative, to nourish the nerves, and to treat states of nervous exhaustion, debility and fatigue, including chronic fatigue syndrome. Oats are excellent in periods of convalescence and when your nerves seem to be under strain, or when you feel weak and in need of support. Oats have been used to support people undergoing drug withdrawal, including from cigarettes, and they provide a gentle, reliable and safe foundation when we are in states of utter exhaustion or complete upheaval.

In addition to taking oats and oat bran as porridge you can take an oatstraw tincture. This is best taken as the 1:1 tincture at a dose of 5–10ml per day in water.

## Passionflower

Despite its name, passionflower (*Passiflora incarnata*) is valued for its abilities to calm and relax nervous energies rather than to rouse them! The name is thought to refer to the Passion of Our Lord because of the association between the appearance of the central part of the flower and the Crown of Thorns. In any event, the flowers are stunning and this climbing plant graces any garden.

245

This is a good herb to take if experiencing periods of hyperactivity, restlessness and difficulty in sleeping. It appears to have a deep nourishing effect on the nerves, helping to improve emotional strength and resilience. If your mind is agitated and you are experiencing chaotic thoughts and indecision, passionflower can help to bring clarity and perspective. Passionflower has a substantial feel to it in terms of its impact on the nervous system, helping us to become anchored and providing us with a breathing space to hone our focus and make changes in direction. This is a herb that will often provide support at life's turning points.

The aerial parts of the plant are used (leaves, stems, flowers) and are prepared as a tea by infusion. Two teaspoons of the herb is used per cup and 2–3 cups per day can be taken. Passionflower combines well with skullcap (*Scutellaria lateriflora*) or St John's wort (*Hypericum perforatum*).

## St John's wort

St John's wort (*Hypericum perforatum*) is so called because it flowers around the time of 'St John's tide' – the Christian renaming of the summer solstice. Earlier peoples of the British Isles and the European mainland held this herb sacred. Among the reasons for this could be that the yellow, sun-like flowers appear at the summer solstice when the sun is at its height, and that the flowers and leaves of this plant are dotted with oil glands which release a pigment when crushed between the fingers that is the colour of blood.

St John's wort has been demonstrated to be effective in treating states of mild to moderate depression and it is widely used for this purpose. It is an excellent herb for depressed states, sadness, despondency, and for when we feel blank and uninspired. It has a nurturing quality and it stabilises our mood when we experience unpleasant fluctuations in our feelings. It is very good for mood changes associated with the menopause and it may also help reduce hot flushes. St John's wort seems to help soothe frayed nerves in nervous exhaustion states and is a great herb for treating 'burnout', when we cease to be able to cope with strain, guiding us back to our former optimism and vitality. Traditionally, St John's wort was taken to treat wounds, all types of bleeding, diarrhoea, jaundice, bladder and kidney problems, and chest infections. Studies have shown that this plant has antiviral properties, especially against the herpes virus group.

St John's wort is a safe and widely applicable herb, but its use is limited by the type of conventional medication that you might also be taking. It speeds up the detoxification of some drugs by the liver so that it can reduce their therapeutic activity, potentially exposing you to risk.

St John's wort can be taken as a tea made by infusion at a dose of 2 teaspoons of the dried whole herb (leaf, stems and flowers) to a cup, with 2–4 cups taken each day. It combines well with skullcap as a supportive, enhancing and strengthening nervous-system tea.

### Caution

There are cautions concerning consuming some conventional drugs at the same time as St John's wort, the most important of which applies to drugs (especially cyclosporin) taken by transplant patients to prevent their body rejecting the transplanted organ. If you are taking conventional medication, you are advised to talk to both your doctor and an experienced herbalist before taking St John's wort.

## Skullcap

Although there is very little research to support its use, skullcap (*Scutellaria lateriflora*) is one of the most revered and frequently prescribed nervines by British herbalists. This may be because it is very safe and well tolerated by a wide range of people, as well as because of its reliable effectiveness in supporting and lifting the mood. Skullcap is a nervous trophorestorative suitable for treating nervous fatigue, and it is also gently calming for states of anxiety and overstimulation. This herb suits people who are highly stressed, uptight and hyperactive. It also seems to relax the perspective of those who maintain set and rigid views which are holding back their human development.

*Scutellaria* derives its name from the Latin for 'a little dish' and it refers to the form of the upper part of the delicate, lilac-purple flowers. The common name continues with the image of the dish and relates it to the type of cap worn by monks. Whatever the origin, the common name is apt as this is very much a herb of quiet contemplation and spiritual growth. Skullcap is a useful herb to take to help us learn from our experiences and it can be especially well suited when attempting to work on your spiritual side.

Skullcap tea is prepared by infusion at a dose of 2 teaspoons of the aerial parts of the plant (stem, leaves and flowers) to a cup. Take 2–4 cups a day.

## Valerian

Valerian (*Valeriana officinalis*) is one of the most useful herbs to combat the effects of stress. It relaxes both the mind and the muscles, having a calming and balancing influence on the nervous system. It is excellent for soothing the nerves in tense situations, for example before taking an examination or giving a performance. It is also helpful where stress tends to cause tension headaches or where stress helps to exacerbate high blood pressure. Irritability, restlessness, insomnia and states of excess energy can also benefit from treatment with valerian. If you are prone to experiencing a tense, explosive reaction to stressful situations, losing your temper easily, becoming overactive and then finding it hard to calm down again, then valerian may be the herb for you. It can also be used for less pronounced reactions. Overall, valerian is a herb that can calm anger and overstimulation, reduce the disquieting background 'chatter' of repetitive irritating thoughts, and help us to focus our mental and emotional energies on more positive issues.

The root of valerian is used as a tea made by decoction at a dose of 1–3g of root per cup, with up to 3 cups taken per day. To aid sleep, take the final cup just before going to bed. Although valerian is a safe and reliable herb, it can occasionally cause an adverse fluctuation in energy levels, either exacerbating tiredness or increasing nervous stimulation. Traditionally, valerian has been taken with other herbs to reduce the small chance of such a side effect. To this end, valerian combines well with skullcap, chamomile or St John's wort. A favourite combination of mine is to use 1 teaspoon of valerian root with 1 teaspoon of skullcap herb to a cup, making the tea by decoction.

The smell of valerian is quite distinctive. To me it is redolent of medieval apothecary shops, but not everyone appreciates it. Cats go crazy over it, so you might want to keep your valerian root in a cupboard where the cat isn't able to roll all over it!

## Vervain

Vervain (*Verbena officinalis*) is another herb that was once held sacred in the British Isles. It is a most attractive plant sending up thin spikes of tiny, pale lilac flowers. It is a marvellous herb to take as a trophorestorative for depletion of the nervous system, during periods of convalescence, and when motivation and energy levels are low. Vervain has a bitter taste which contributes to its tonic effect by stimulating the liver and the digestive system. Traditionally, the liver was said to be the seat of melancholy and bitter nervines, which could reduce congestion of the liver, were much prized. Vervain has a strong, deep, transforming and grounding influence on the emotional state. It helps to reduce fear, nightmares and confused states, bringing calm, clarity and confidence. Although vervain can benefit both men and women, it has a long tradition in helping nervous-system changes in women such as the mood disturbances associated with premenstrual syndrome and the menopause.

Vervain leaves on their own or the whole herb (leaves, stems and flowers) are used medicinally. A tea is made by infusion at a dose of 1–2 teaspoons of the herb per cup, with up to 3 cups taken daily. Because of its bitterness it can be helpful to combine vervain with lemon balm at a dose of 1 teaspoon of each herb per cup. During breast-feeding, a combination of vervain and borage at a dose of 1 teaspoon of each per cup can be taken as both herbs encourage milk flow and help the nervous system to cope with the stress of parenthood. I have also seen good results in several cases of post-natal depression using this combination.

## KEY HERB FOR THE MIND AND EMOTIONS

## LEMON BALM

**Scientific name** *Melissa officinalis*

**Plant family** Lamiaceae (mint family)

**Type of plant** Perennial herb.

**Part used** Leaves.

**Phytochemicals** Rosmarinic acid, volatile oil.

**Actions** Antioxidant, antispasmodic, antiviral, cardiac sedative, carminative, diaphoretic, mood enhancer

**Indications** Lemon balm is generally helpful for improving mood and also as part of the treatment of cold sores (herpes virus infection around the mouth; in this case lemon balm is applied topically to the sore), depression, fevers, high blood pressure, indigestion and irritable bowel syndrome. There is also an association with improving memory and extending longevity.

**Preparations** The tea is made by infusing 2 teaspoons of the dried herb and it can be taken 1–4 times a day. A tincture made from the fresh herb at a strength of 1:2 in 45% alcohol can be taken at a dose of 4–8ml per day in water.

**Combinations** Lemon balm combines well with limeflowers for treating angina and high blood pressure, and with passionflower as a general soothing tea for the nervous system.

**Cautions** May occasionally accentuate high moods, causing euphoria and restlessness, and should therefore be avoided in excited states of joy and delight.

**Conservation** Lemon balm is easily cultivated and poses no environmental concerns. It is native to southern Europe, western Asia and north Africa, but can occasionally be seen growing in the wild in the UK as a garden escapee.

# APPENDIX – THE SYNDROME X DIET

## Stage 1

For 2 weeks, cut out the following foods completely, using the substitutes suggested instead. This avoids high glycaemic index foods and foods that negatively influence blood sugar levels.

| Do not eat | Do eat |
|---|---|
| Flour products (white and brown) – bread, baguettes, crackers, pastries, pasta, spaghetti, etc. Read packets so that you avoid wheat added to other products. | Eat a variety of grains such as brown rice, millet, barley, quinoa, and pulses such as red kidney beans, chick peas, haricot beans, butter beans, aduki beans, lentils. Instead of wheat crackers try rice cakes. |
| Sugar (white and brown) – do not add sugar to food or drinks. | Get used to hot drinks and foods without sugar added. |
| Chocolate, boiled sweets, chewing gum, toffee, nougat, cakes, buns, mints. | Fruit – all sorts, especially the strongly antioxidant fruits such as: apples, apricots, blackcurrants, cherries, bilberries, blueberries, grapes (red, black), grapefruit, oranges, satsumas, tangerines, clementines and strawberries. |

| Do not eat | Do eat |
| --- | --- |
| | Vegetables – as snacks, such as raw carrots and celery. |
| Crisps, chips, deep-fried foods. | Nuts – Brazils, walnuts, cashews, pine nuts, hazelnuts. Seeds – sesame, pumpkin, sunflower. |
| Hard cheese, dairy milk. | Cottage cheese, soya or rice milk. |
| Coffee (including decaffeinated) – this leads to peaks and troughs in blood sugar levels and stimulates sugar cravings. | Use caffeine-free substitutes such as dandelion coffee and those based on barley and chicory. |
| China and Indian tea (and speciality teas based on these) – like coffee, also interferes with sugar levels though not as strongly. Tannins in tea prevent absorption of nutrients such as selenium that balance sugar levels in the blood. | Rooibos (red bush) tea, Mountain honeybush tea. Use herbal teas but avoid 'fruit teas' – try chamomile, fennel, elderflower, peppermint, hawthorn, nettle. |
| Fruit juices – even fresh, home-pressed juices have very high sugar levels. | 'Smoothies' with whole fruit and natural yoghurt – include peels where appropriate (fruit peels contain soluble fibre that mops up sugar). |
| Honey, maple syrup, date syrup, blackstrap molasses, golden syrup and other natural sweeteners need to be avoided. | No substitute – you need to lose your craving for sweet tastes. It may sound hard but you need to learn to enjoy the natural taste |

| Do not eat | Do eat |
|---|---|
| | of foods without sugar enhancers. |
| Artificial sweeteners should be avoided – they are not a healthy alternative to sugar. | There is no need to substitute these – they are an anti-nutrient. |
| Fizzy drinks – keep away from cola drinks, glucose drinks, 'sports' and similar drinks. Also, squashes should be avoided. | Mineral water. Still water is preferable but use sparkling if you really want the fizz effect. |
| Peanut butter. | Tahini (sesame seed spread); cashew nut butter; almond butter. |

*To complement Stage 1 and enhance detoxification avoid all alcohol for the 2 weeks.*

Although this may look difficult at first, after 2 weeks you should find that your cravings subside and it becomes easy to resist temptation.

## Stage 2

After 2 weeks, follow these guidelines as part of your everyday dietary regime.

### Your Healthy Diet Plan

• Slowly bring back wholemeal flour products such as bread and pasta (pasta is made of durum wheat, which releases sugars into the body more slowly than other wheat products; it can therefore be taken occasionally). Continue to avoid white flour products completely and make wholemeal flour products a balanced element of the diet – do not consume them several times a day every day.

- Continue to eat whole grains (other than wheat) and pulses. It is good to vary these so that you have a different type of grain each day or so in rotation. Eat grains and pulses together (or within 24 hours of each other) as this enhances protein variety and uptake.

- Introduce oatcakes into your diet, in addition to rice cakes, but only in moderation. Continue to avoid wheat crackers.

- Bring in cheese and dairy milk in moderation. Do not have cheese every day; do not drink whole glasses of dairy milk. Use cottage cheese in preference to hard cheese. Use soya milk and rice milk wherever possible.

- Eat natural live yoghurt – flavour with chopped fresh fruit.

- Add soya products to the diet – especially tofu and tempeh.

- Continue to avoid honey, maple syrup and other natural sweeteners. Use dried fruit to sweeten such foods as porridge and cakes for special occasions, but do not use such these every day.

- Never, ever use packet sugar again – refined, raw cane or otherwise. Do not have it in the house. Remember, it can make you ill and shorten your life.

- Eat plenty of vegetable-based meals. Keep your fruit and vegetable intake high.

- Continue to avoid chocolate, boiled sweets, chewing gum, toffee, nougat, cakes, buns and mints with a firm resolve; these substances can be toxic for you.

- For snacks, eat fruit, raw vegetables, nuts and seeds – for a more filling snack use raw vegetable sticks with a hummus dip.

- Plan ahead – if you are going out, ensure you have a fruit/vegetable/nut/seed snack with you – carry them with you, and leave some at work. Do not get caught out!

- Try to keep off coffee and tea, but, if necessary, keep them as occasional treats rather than day-to-day beverages.

- Eat potatoes (especially baked), but do not have them every day. Just as it is important to eat a variety of grains, it is essential to eat a variety of vegetables.

- Do not go too long without eating. Remember to have breakfast – porridge or muesli is better than toast. Remember that the best snacks for you are fruit, nuts and seeds.

- Do not go for more than an hour without drinking. Make water your main drink, together with some rooibos, barley and rye drinks, and herbal teas.

- Bring back alcohol if you wish but stick to the following guidelines. Red wine, cider and whisky (12-year-old single malts) all contain antioxidant polyphenols which may have beneficial effects on health (protecting against heart disease and cancer) but only when taken as below:

  - Only drink with food – avoid drinking on an empty stomach; drink while eating and up to half an hour before to one and a half hours after meals;

  - Have 2 days a week with no alcohol intake at all;

  - For 5 days a week drink 1–3 glasses of red wine per day;

  - For every measure of alcohol, drink an equal amount of water soon afterwards;

  - Drink little and often rather than large amounts infrequently;

  - Do not mix drinks.

# GLOSSARY OF HERB NAMES

| | |
|---|---|
| Agrimony | *Agrimonia eupatorium* |
| Allspice | *Pimenta dioica* |
| Angelica | *Angelica archangelica* |
| Aniseed | *Pimpinella anisum* |
| Ashwagandha (winter cherry, 'Indian ginseng') | *Withania somnifera* |
| Baical Skullcap | *Scutellaria baicalensis* |
| Basil | *Ocimum* species |
| Beetroot | *Beta vulgaris* |
| Bilberry | *Vaccinium myrtillus* |
| Birch | *Betula* species |
| Blackberry | *Rubus fruticosus* |
| Black cohosh | *Cimicifuga racemosa* |
| Black haw | *Viburnum prunifolium* |
| Black pepper | *Piper nigrum* |
| Black walnut | *Juglans nigra* |
| Blue gum | *Eucalyptus globulus* |
| Boldo | *Peumus boldus* |
| Boneset | *Eupatorium perfoliatum* |
| Borage | *Borago officinalis* |
| Buckwheat | *Fagopyrum esculentum* |
| Burdock | *Arctium lappa* |
| Butternut | *Juglans cinerea* |

| | |
|---|---|
| Californian poppy | *Eschscholzia californica* |
| Canadian (American) ginseng | *Panax quinquefolius* |
| Caraway | *Carum carvi* |
| Carrots | *Daucus carota* |
| Cascara sagrada | *Rhamnus purshiana* |
| Cat's claw | *Uncaria tomentosa* |
| Celery | *Apium graveolens* |
| Centaury | *Centaurium erythrea* |
| Chamomile | *Matricaria recutita* (*Chamomilla recutita*) |
| Chasteberry | *Vitex agnus-castus* |
| Chilli peppers | *Capsicum* species |
| Chinese magnolia vine (Wu Wei Zi) | *Schisandra chinensis* |
| Chiretta | *Andrographis paniculata* |
| Chives | *Allium schoenoprasum* |
| Cinnamon | *Cinnamomum zeylanicum* |
| Cleavers | *Galium aparine* |
| Cloves | *Syzygium aromaticum* |
| Coca | *Erythroxylum coca* |
| Cola | *Cola nitida* |
| Coltsfoot | *Tussilago farfara* |
| Couch grass | *Elymus repens* |
| Cramp bark (Guelder rose) | *Viburnum opulus* |
| Cumin | *Cuminum cyminum* |
| Damiana | *Turnera diffusa* |
| Dan Shen | *Salvia miltiorrhiza* |
| Dandelion | *Taraxacum officinale* |
| Devil's claw | *Harpagophytum procumbens* |
| Devil's club | *Oplopanax horridus* |
| Dill | *Anethum graveolens* |
| Dong quai (Chinese ginseng, 'women's ginseng') | *Angelica sinensis* |
| East Indian walnut | *Albizia lebbeck* |

| | |
|---|---|
| Echinacea (coneflower) | *Echinacea purpurea* |
| Elderflower | *Sambucus nigra* |
| Elecampane | *Inula hellenium* |
| Eucalyptus | *Eucalyptus* species |
| Evening primrose | *Oenethera biennis* |
| Fennel | *Foeniculum vulgare* |
| Fenugreek | *Trigonella foenum-graecum* |
| Feverfew | *Tanacetum parthenium* |
| Figwort | *Scrophularia nodosa* |
| Frankincense | *Boswellia sacra* |
| Fumitory | *Fumaria officinalis* |
| Garlic | *Allium sativum* |
| Ginger | *Zingiber officinale* |
| Gingko | *Gingko biloba* |
| Globe artichoke | *Cynara scolymus* |
| Goat's rue | *Galega officinalis* |
| Golden rod | *Solidago virgaurea* |
| Golden seal | *Hydrastis canadensis* |
| Gotu cola (gotu kola) | *Centella asiatica (Hydrocotyle asiatica)* |
| Grape | *Vitis vinifera* |
| Ground ivy | *Glechoma hederacea* |
| Guarana ('Brazilian ginseng') | *Paullinia cupana* |
| Gully gum | *Eucalyptus smithii* |
| Gum arabic | *Acacia senegal* |
| Gumplant | *Grindelia camporum* |
| Gurmar | *Gymnema sylvestre* |
| Hare's ear (Chai Hu) | *Bupleurum falcatum* |
| Hawthorn | *Crataegus* species |
| He Shou Wu | *Polygonum multiflorum* |
| Hemp | *Cannabis sativa* |
| Hops | *Humulus lupulus* |
| Horse chestnut | *Aesculus hippocastanum* |
| Horseradish | *Armoracia rusticana* |

| | |
|---|---|
| Houseleeks | *Sempervivum* species |
| Hyssop | *Hyssopus officinalis* |
| Ipecac | *Cephaelis ipecacaunha* |
| Jamaica dogwood | *Piscidia erythrina* |
| Kava | *Piper methysticum* |
| Knitbone (Comfrey) | *Symphytum officinale* |
| Korean Ginseng | *Panax ginseng* |
| (Asiatic Ginseng) | |
| Lavender | *Lavandula angustifolia* |
| Leek | *Allium ampeloprasum* |
| Lemon balm | *Melissa officinalis* |
| Lesser periwinkle | *Vinca minor* |
| Lily of the valley | *Convallaria majalis* |
| Lime | *Tilia* species |
| Linseed | *Linum usitatissimum* |
| Liquorice | *Glycyrrhiza glabra* |
| Lovage | *Levisticum officinale* |
| Ma huang | *Ephedra sinica* |
| Maize (corn) | *Zea mays* |
| Marigold | *Calendula officinalis* |
| Maritime pine | *Pinus pinaster* (*Pinus maritima*) |
| Marsh cudweed | *Gnaphalium uliginosum* |
| Marshmallow | *Althaea officinalis* |
| Mastic | *Pistacia lentiscus* |
| Meadowsweet | *Filipendula ulmaria* |
| Milk thistle | *Silybum marianum* |
| (St Mary's Thistle) | (*Carduus marianus*) |
| Milk vetch | *Astragalus membranaceus* |
| Motherwort | *Leonurus cardiaca* |
| Muira puama | *Ptychopetalum olacoides* |
| Mullein | *Verbascum thapsus* |
| Myrrh | *Commiphora molmol* |
| Nasturtium | *Tropaeolum majus* |
| Neem | *Azadirachta indica* |

| | |
|---|---|
| Nettle | *Urtica dioica* |
| Oak, common | *Quercus robur* |
| Oats | *Avena sativa* |
| Olive | *Olea europea* |
| Onion | *Allium cepa* |
| Opium poppy | *Papaver somniferum* |
| Oregano | *Origanum* species |
| Oregon grape | *Mahonia aquifolium* (*Berberis aquifolium*) |
| Parsley piert | *Aphanes arvensis* |
| Passionflower | *Passiflora incarnata* |
| Pau d'arco | *Tabebuia* species |
| Pellitory-of-the-wall | *Parietaria judaica* (*Parietaria diffusa*) |
| Peppermint | *Mentha piperita* |
| Psyllium | *Plantago psyllium* |
| Quassia | *Picrasma excelsa* |
| Raspberry | *Rubus idaeus* |
| Red clover | *Trifolium pratense* |
| Reishi | *Ganoderma lucidum* |
| Rhubarb | *Rheum palmatum* |
| Ribwort plantain | *Plantago lanceolata* |
| Rooibos (rooibosch, red bush) | *Aspalanthus linearis* |
| Rose | *Rosa damascena* |
| Rose root (golden root, Arctic root) | *Rhodiola rosea* |
| Rosemary | *Rosmarinus officinalis* |
| Sage | *Salvia officinalis* |
| Salai guggal | *Boswellia serrata* |
| Sandalwood | *Santalum album* |
| Sarsaparilla | *Smilax* species |
| Saw palmetto | *Serenoa serulata* |
| Skullcap | *Scutellaria lateriflora* |
| Sheep's sorrel | *Rumex acetosella* |

| | |
|---|---|
| Siberian ginseng | *Eleutherococcus senticosus* |
| Slippery elm | *Ulmus rubra* (*Ulmus fulva*) |
| Spearmint | *Mentha spicata* |
| Spruce | *Picea* species |
| St John's wort | *Hypericum perforatum* |
| Stonecrop | *Sedum* species |
| Sweet almond | *Prunus dulcis* |
| Sweet flag | *Acorus calamus* |
| Sweet potato | *Ipomoea batatas* |
| Sweet violet | *Viola odorata* |
| Tea | *Camellia sinensis* |
| Thornapple | *Datura stramonium* |
| Thyme | *Thymus vulgaris* |
| Turmeric | *Curcuma longa* |
| Valerian | *Valeriana officinalis* |
| Vervain | *Verbena officinalis* |
| Walnut, English | *Juglans regia* |
| Watercress | *Nasturtium officinale* |
| White horehound | *Marrubium vulgare* |
| Wild cherry | *Prunus serotina* |
| Wild garlic (ransoms) | *Allium ursinum* |
| Wild yam | *Dioscorea villosa* |
| Willow | *Salix* species |
| Witch hazel | *Hamamelis virginiana* |
| Wormwood | *Artemisia absinthium* |
| Yarrow | *Achillea millefolium* |
| Yellow dock | *Rumex crispus* |

# FURTHER READING

Ashton J. and Laura R., *The Perils of Progress: the Health and Environment Hazards of Modern Technology, and What You Can Do About Them*, Zed Books, 1998

Balick M. and Cox P., *Plants, People and Culture: the Science of Ethnobotany*, Scientific American Library, 1997

Barker J., *The Medicinal Flora of Britain and Northwestern Europe*, Winter Press, 2001

Bartram T., *Encyclopaedia of Herbal Medicine*, Grace, 1995

Bensky D. and Gamble A., *Chinese Herbal Medicine Materia Medica*, Eastland Press, 1993

BHMA, *British Herbal Pharmacopoeia*, British Herbal Medicine Association, 1983

Boik J., *Natural Compounds in Cancer Therapy*, Oregon Medical Press, 2001

Bone K., *Clinical Applications of Ayurvedic and Chinese Herbs*, Phytotherapy Press, 1996

Chaitow L., *Principles of Fasting*, Thorsons, 1996

Chevallier A., *The Encyclopaedia of Medicinal Plants*, Dorling Kindersley, 1996

Conway P., *Tree Medicine*, Piatkus, 2001

Cook Wm. H., *The Physio-Medical Dispensatory*, Wm. H. Cook Eclectic Medical Publications, 1985

Corrigan D., *Gingko Biloba: Ancient Medicine*, Amberwood, 1995

Devaraj T.L., *Speaking of Ayurvedic Remedies for Common Diseases*, Sterling, 1994

Ellingwood F., *American Materia Medica, Therapeutics and Pharmacognosy*, Eclectic Medical Publications, 1994

Fulder S., *The Root of Being: Ginseng and the Pharmacology of Harmony*, Hutchinson, 1980

Grieve M., *A Modern Herbal*, Tiger, 1992

Griggs B., *New Green Pharmacy*, Vermillion, 1997

Griggs B., *Reinventing Eden*, Quadrille, 2001

Groombridge B. and Jenkins M.D., *Global Biodiversity: Earth's Living Resources in the 21st Century*, World Conservation Press, 2000

Guyton A.C. and Hall J.E., *Textbook of Medical Physiology*, W.B. Saunders & Co, 2000

Hatfield G., *Memory, Wisdom and Healing: the History of Domestic Plant Medicine*, Sutton, 1999

Kaptchuk T.J., *Chinese Medicine: the Web That Has No Weaver*, Rider, 1983

Lloyd G.E.R. (ed), *Hippocratic Writings*, Penguin, 1978

Mabberley D.J., *The Plant Book*, Cambridge University Press, 1987

Mills S. and Bone K., *Principles and Practice of Phytotherapy – Modern Herbal Medicine*, Churchill Livingstone, 2000

Moerman D.E., *Native American Ethnobotany*, Timber Press, 1998

Murray M.T., *The Healing Power of Herbs*, Prima, 1995

Nadkarni A.K., *Indian Materia Medica*, Popular Prakashan, 1954

Pengelly A., *The Constituents of Medicinal Plants*, Sunflower Herbals, 1997

Pizzorno J.E. and Murray M.T., *Textbook of Natural Medicine*, Churchill Livingstone, 1999

Porter R., *The Greatest Benefit to Mankind – a Medical History of Humanity from Antiquity to the Present Day*, HarperCollins, 1997

Priest A.W. and Priest L.R., *Herbal Medication*, C.W. Daniel/National Institute of Medical Herbalists, 2000

Weiss R.F. and Fintelmann V., *Herbal Medicine*, Thieme, 2000

Wren R.C., *Potter's New Cyclopaedia of Botanical Drugs and Preparations*, C.W. Daniel, 1988

Zimmermann M., *Burgerstein's Handbook of Nutrition*, Thieme, 2001

# RESOURCES

## Books

### Cooking

The following are recommended as they help to plan meals that contain antioxidant fruits, vegetables, nuts, seeds and soya products.

Bates D.R., *The Tempeh Cookbook*, Book Publishing Co, 1989
Clark S., *Moro: The Cookbook*, Ebury Press, 2001
Freed H., *Eating in Eden*, Rudra Press, 1998
Greenberg P. and Newton Hartung H., *The Whole Soy Cookbook*, Three Rivers Press, 1998
Leneman L., *The Tofu Cookbook*, HarperCollins, 1998
Wakeman A. and Baskerville G., *The Vegan Cookbook*, Faber and Faber, 1996

### Growing herbs

De la Bedoyere C., *How to Grow Culinary Herbs and Spices the Natural Way*, HDRA/Search Press, 1994
Rees Y. and Titterington R., *Growing Herbs*, Aura Books, 1994

# Useful Addresses
## Growing herbs
*Biodynamic Agricultural Association*
Painswick Inn, Stroud
Gloucestershire, UK
Tel: 01453 759501
Web site: bdaa@biodynamic.freeserve.co.uk
E-mail: www.anth.org.uk/biodynamic

*Biodynamic Farming and Gardening Association*
Building 1002B, Thoreau Centre
The Presidio, PO Box 29315
San Francisco, CA USA
Web site: biodynamic@aol.com
E-mail: www.biodynamics.com

*Soil Association*
Bristol House, 40–56 Victoria Street
Bristol, BS1 6BY, UK
Tel: 0117 929 0661
Web site: info@soilassociation.org
E-mail: www.soilassociation.org

*Herbs in Australia*
Web site: www.oldvegiepatch.netfirms.com/herb.htm
E-mail: greenpaddocks@mydesk.net.au

*Herb Federation of New Zealand*
PO Box 280
Waihi, New Zealand
E-mail: herbfederationnewzealand@xtra.co.nz

*Botanical Society of South Africa*
Private Bag X 10
Claremount 7735, South Africa
Web site: www.botanicalsociety.org.za
E-mail: info@botanicalsociety.org.za

## Herbal suppliers

Napier's Direct
35 Hamilton Place
Edinburgh, EH3 5BA, UK

Tel: 0131 343 6683
Web site: webmaster@napiers.net
E-mail: www.napiers.net

Napier's herbal dispensary is a famous and long-established herbal house in Scotland. The details above are for its mail order branch, which offers a wide range of herbal products.

*Neal's Yard Remedies*
29 John Dalton Street
Manchester, M2 6DS, UK

Tel: 0161 8317875
Web site: mailorder@nealsyardremedies.com

A well-established herbal supplier.

*The Organic Herb Trading Company*
Milverton, Somerset, TA4 1NF, UK

Tel: 01823 – 401205.
Web site: www.organicherbtrading.com

This company supplies medicinal herbs, tinctures and oils, specialising in those that have been grown organically.

*Gaia Garden Herbal Apothecary*
2672 West Broadway
Vancouver BC
Canada V6K 2G3
Web site: www.gaiagarden.com

## Herbal practitioner registers

*American Herbalists Guild*
1931 Gaddis Road, Canton

GA 30115, USA

Web site: www.healthy.net/herbalists/

The AHS holds a list of approved herbal practitioners in the US.

*College of Practitioners of Phytotherapy*
Marley Lane
Battle, East Sussex, TN33 0TY

One of the major professional organisations for herbal medicine in the UK. Provides a list of qualified phytotherapists.

*National Herbalists Association of Australia*
NHAA, P.O. Box 61, Broadway
NSW 2007, Australia

Web site: www.nhaa.org.au

The NHAA was founded in 1920 and provides details of qualified herbalists in Australia.

*National Institute of Medical Herbalists*
56 Longbrook Street, Exeter
Devon EX4 6AH, UK

Tel: 01392 426022

Web site: www.btinternet.com/~nimh/

Established in 1864, this is the main professional body for medical herbalists in the UK. They can provide details of training courses in herbal medicine and a directory of qualified practitioners. This website contains listings of practitioners around the world.

*Ontario Herbalists Association*
RR 1
Port Burwell
Ontario, Canada N0J 1T0

Web site: www.herbalists.on.ca

E-mail: fieldofdaisies@canada.com

# INDEX

Note: page numbers in **bold** refer to major references to herbs.

secondary metabolites 15–16
sedatives 243, 244–6, 248–9, 251
seeds 36
selective estrogen receptor
    modulators (SERMs) 223
selenium 89, 115, 189, 191, 192,
    219, 224
self-esteem 216
self-healing 23
self-treatment 12–13, 27–8
Siberian ginseng (*Eleutherococcus
    senticosus*) **47**, 59, **98–9**,
    **102–3, 108–9**, 217, 239
skin 73–4, 185–202
    dry 190
    tone 193
skullcap (*Scutellaria lateriflora*) 34,
    196, **248**
sleep 116, 235
slippery elm (*Ulmus rubra*) 18, 136,
    143–4
smoking 53, 74–5, 156, 173
smoothies 254
soya 208, 256
spearmint (*Mentha spicata*) 177
sperm 84
spiritual purification 69
standardised extracts 29–31
steam inhalation 178–9
stimulants 159–60, 164, 195, 217,
    238–9
stomach 130
stomach ulcers 84, 130, 140
storing herbs 32, 37
stress 116, 119, 156–7
sugary foods 50, 51, 154, 253, 254,
    256
sunlight 188
superbugs ix, 111
sweat lodges 73
sweet almond oil (*Prunus dulcis*)
    179
sweet corn (*Zea mays*) 73
sweet flag (*Acorus calamus*) 136

sweet violet (*Viola odorata*) 75, 177
Syndrome X (Insulin Resistance
    Syndrome) 151–2, 160–1, 212
Syndrome X Diet xii, 50, 157, 162,
    253–7

tablets 41, 43
tannins 19–20, 85, 86, 134, 254
taste of herbs 21, 32
tea
    black 52, 90–1, 134, 254, 256
    detoxing 54, 61, 64, 77–8
    green 90–1, 134
    herbal 38–9, 54, 58, 59, 61, 64,
        77–9, 177–8, 254
    rooibos 91, 134
temperature, atmospheric 56–7
testosterone 223
therapeutic effects of herbs 21
therapeutic window, narrow 25
thornapple (*Datura stramonium*) 16
thyme (*Thymus vulgaris*) 34, 54, 74,
    90, 91, 175, 176, 177, 178, 179,
    **183–4**
tinctures 39, 42, 43
tisanes 38–9
tonics x, 24, 100, 177–8
toxins 66–9, 116, 134
    *see also* environmental toxins
trachea 168–9
Traditional Chinese Medicine
    (TCM) 6–7, 9, 21
training 11
transporting herbs 28
triterpenoid saponins 95
tryptophan 212
turmeric (*Curcuma longa*) 58, 90,
    195, **201**

valerian (*Valeriana officinalis*) xi, 30,
    34, 35, **48**, 138, 160, 196,
    **248–9**
vata 7
vegetables 58, 61, 87–8, 256